SHRINK
THE DIET
FOR THE
MIND

TESTIMONIALS

"Mindful eating saved my life. Seriously! I'm back to size 12 and my pre-children weight. I'm even coping okay with the menopause. I look in the mirror and see the real me, and that's priceless." **SARAH**

"Philippe has had a profound impact on my life. I lost over 13 kilos (2 stone) in about three months. He is straightforward, insightful, kind and his method makes perfect sense. The weight loss feels long lasting because he addresses deep-rooted reasons for overeating as well as changing unhelpful eating patterns and discussing potential stumbling blocks. So many people have told me how great I am looking and have asked me what diet I'm on and I reply, 'It's not a diet – it's Philippe!'" **SUSAN**

"I started work with Philippe on getting my weight down through psychology and thereby taking a holistic approach. It has been hugely successful and what he has helped me with in particular is banishing my mental demons, which leads to improved health and wellbeing. It is a huge relief to get rid of my tiresome baggage, both mentally and physically." **STEVE**

"Working with Philippe has given me new insight and new techniques to address my issues with food and has helped me lose weight without dieting. It's not magic: it requires openness and commitment to be successful but I believe this approach can provide a sustainable answer to my years of yo-yo dieting." **VANESSA**

SHRINK
THE DIET
FOR THE
MIND

Retrain
Your Brain &
Lose Weight
for Good

PHILIPPE TAHON

aster

An Hachette UK Company
www.hachette.co.uk

First published in Great Britain in 2018 by Aster,
an imprint of Octopus Publishing Group Ltd
Carmelite House
50 Victoria Embankment
London EC4Y 0DZ
www.octopusbooks.co.uk

Distributed in the US by Hachette Book Group
1290 Avenue of the Americas, 4th and 5th Floors
New York, NY 10104

Distributed in Canada by Canadian Manda Group
664 Annette St., Toronto, Ontario, Canada M6S 2C8

ISBN 978-1-91202-386-8

A CIP catalogue record for this book is available from the British Library.

Printed and bound by CPI Group (UK) Ltd, Croydon, CR0 4YY

10 9 8 7 6 5 4 3 2 1

Publishing Director: Stephanie Jackson
Art Director: Juliette Norsworthy
Design: The Oak Studio Limited
Cover Design: Aaron Munday
Junior Editor: Ella Parsons
Copy Editor: Steve Gove
Production Controller: Grace O'Byrne

CONTENTS

"If you do not change direction, you may end up where you are heading."

LAOZI, CHINESE PHILOSOPHER, 6TH CENTURY BC

An Open Letter to the Creators and Purveyors of Fad Diets

Dear diet gurus,

I am writing this letter to compliment you on the excellent work you are doing. Indeed, thanks to you, more and more people are seeking my help to lose weight.

The suggestions you make may all look different, but they are ultimately very similar. Between them, they have greatly contributed to removing any nutritional benchmarks for millions of people in distress.

I admire how you manage to convince so many individuals of the merits of your theories: you are the new gurus of those souls in perdition!

But I must admit that you also complicate my task. Thanks to you, my clients want near-instant results and specific instructions to get back their youthful figures. They look at me incredulously when I tell them that I am not going to put them on a diet and that they have to rediscover their food sensations. And they hate it when I warn them that this could take some time...

I understand their scepticism: you have accustomed them to expect immediate results.

We make an unlikely alliance, you and I. You systematically destroy their common sense when it comes to food and make them lose weight so quickly that it will inevitably pile back on in no time at all. I pick up the pieces when, after several attempts at different fads, they are completely disempowered and depressed and many have developed serious eating disorders.

If I wasn't so angry, I'd suggest we go into business together - but then I suspect the medical profession would need to join us too, as they are the ones who have to care for all those with serious health issues after following your methods.

I am doing my best to show them there is another way, but I know that - sadly - I will have my work cut out for years ahead.

But I know, with time, I can help my clients free themselves of the diet trap and achieve life-changing results. It is a challenge I relish.

Philippe Tahon

INTRODUCTION:
TIME FOR CHANGE

"My life revolves around eating. I spend my days thinking about food from the moment I wake up to the minute I fall asleep. It feels like too much effort to lose weight, but Philippe has helped me see that it takes even more effort to stay as I am."

Our relationship with food is intensely intimate and stimulates almost all of our senses. From the day we're born and latch straight onto our mother's breast to receive milk that offers us warmth and comfort, we learn the pleasure of feeding our hunger.

Throughout our lives we receive untold numbers of emotional and physical triggers that compel us to eat, then we consider what we might like by using our senses, before putting food into our mouths, tasting it and swallowing.

Nobody else does that for us. What and how much goes into our digestive system is our responsibility and ours alone. Inevitably, some of what we consume becomes part of us. If we eat too much or too little, then this will actually change what we are, altering our shape, affecting our health and impacting on our mental state.

As a direct result of what and how much they've eaten, every day millions of people look in the mirror and don't like what they see. They may only be a few pounds overweight but, for them, it looks and feels like so much more. Whether they are clinically obese or just a little flabby around the middle, some people can feel trapped in a body they're ashamed of and wracked with guilt about how they allowed themselves to get that way. Many become obsessed with their own self-image from the minute they wake up to the moment they fall asleep. They want to change and have tried numerous diets in the past but feel doomed to fail.

This overwhelming sense of failure is compounded by the way social media, the press and the fashion industry portray what's beautiful and what's ugly. It's further intensified by the way food companies and the sugar lobby advertise their products, associating them with love and happiness. By contrast, gaining weight is associated with laziness, greed and a lack of control. Through millions of lies told every day on television and online, people are subjected to body shaming – especially teenagers.

The multibillion-pound diet industry feeds on these insecure feelings of guilt and self-hatred to lure the desperate into trying every new fad. Advertisements tell us directly or indirectly that we have no willpower and that we are in need of help. They promise that they have a quick and simple answer – the solution to our problems. All we have to do is eat this or drink that, try this new regime or take that concoction. Foolishly, we believe them and hope that this diet will be "the one".

> **"I weigh myself at least twenty times a day. If I think I'm even half a pound too heavy even after I've gone to the toilet and had my shower, I blow-dry my hair in the hope it will make a difference."**

One of the first things I do whenever I meet a new client is ask them how they feel about their own body. Day in day out, I hear people confess that they feel condemned to live in a body they don't recognize, or that they even reject.

They have become unhealthily fixated on what they look like and what others think of them. Having tried almost every diet in the past, they've finally come to appreciate that they need to look more deeply into their relationship with food and their obsessions with how they look. They have heard that I can help.

Many tell me that the minute they wake up they run their hands down their body to see if they can feel their hipbones and have lost weight in the night. Even more confess to critically studying their reflections in mirrors and shop windows. At war with their own bodies, clients like these are locked in a toxic cycle: upset and angry with themselves and bitterly disappointed with the new "miracle diet" that promised to make them thin.

"I love food too much," they lament, or, "I've got no willpower." It was something I used to tell myself crossly during the years that I was overweight too, not realizing that this concept of helplessness in the face of overriding odds neatly absolved me from all personal responsibility.

My clients then bombard me with questions about what they should or shouldn't be eating or how many steps they should be walking each day, all the while complaining that they'll never reach their (often unrealistic) target weight. Judging themselves through the false prism of the glossy images they see on television, on social media or in magazines, many of them are not, in fact, grossly overweight at all. Instead, they are suffering from body dysmorphic disorder where they believe they're much larger than they really are, or think that parts of their bodies are "disgusting" or "hideous".

A surprising number are also tormented by a relatively new condition known as orthorexia nervosa, in which they fixate on what they eat and develop obsessive, anxious behaviour in pursuit of a healthier diet. Whether they have this condition or not, many will seek to control their weight by any means.

I've even heard female clients declare that they will never have children, because "I'll get fat and ugly and my body will never be the same again." It is so sad when people deny themselves one of the greatest joys in life – bringing a new human being into this world – because they are too afraid of the physical consequences. Trying to reassure them, I say, "Where is it written, please, that you can't be slim again after pregnancy? You are a very determined woman who knows what she wants. Why would that change?"

It is true that pregnancy is often a defining moment in the history of a woman's weight gain, and it is not uncommon for women to have a hard time losing that weight after pregnancy. Coupled with hormonal changes this can sometimes become the trigger for things to get worse afterward.

What I am able to show clients is that, even though pregnancy is a time when emotions and cravings are awakened, it is still possible to apply the principles of mindfulness to eating – in other words, taking the time to question how hungry we are, savouring what we eat, and stopping once we are full. The important thing is that we pay attention to what we are feeling, learn how to accept those emotions, talk about them, and move on.

———————————

Many women also feel as if they have completely lost touch with all their usual habits and rituals after giving birth, especially if their eating habits were very different during pregnancy. Add fatigue to the equation and food can often feel like an easy fix, although good management of exhaustion would make a far healthier option. Whatever emotions and feelings come to the fore, it is essential to trust yourself and accept that this is only temporary. Things will return to normal after time has passed and once you learn how to be more mindful, which I will show you how to do in the following chapters.

Another problem for some new mothers is that after giving birth they no longer see themselves as a woman but only as a mother, which in turn can somehow psychologically legitimize their extra weight. This may actually suit them for a while because losing their "baby weight" can spark a kind of mourning for the intimacy and joy of pregnancy, but it will eventually become cumbersome.

I invite these clients to reconnect with the woman inside them and accept their desire to be a healthier size. So many of them no longer feel sexually desirable and even refuse the advances of their husband or partner for the same reasons. This too can be a way of staying in the special emotional cocoon they have created for themselves and their infant.

Once again, I help remind them that they have gone through enormous changes and it will take time for them to rediscover themselves.

My role is to guide all of my clients – and you – through this process until you not only believe that things can be different but actually start to see the changes happening before your eyes. These profound changes can be life-altering and finally allow you to be the person you secretly want to be, rather than conforming to the negative image you have of yourself.

"Each morning I'd eat a bowl of cereal while waiting for my toast, which I slathered with butter and marmalade. That was my routine. I ate it so fast I didn't even stop to think if I really needed to eat that much first thing."

Only when we take time to fully consider the reasons why we eat and when, can we finally allow ourselves to enjoy food for the pleasure that it is. Once we've mastered this, a love of cooking and enjoying tasty healthy meals becomes a plus not a minus. I know this because I used to own restaurants and I've always loved to cook for myself and for friends and family. Deciding what to make and creating something from scratch can empower us to regain control of our diet and encourage us to reconnect with food in a positive, healthy way.

I have clients who lose all the weight they wanted with my help and then keep on losing it, beyond their target. They sometimes ask me, "When will the weight loss stop?", looking to me for further guidance.

Instead I laugh and say, "It will stop whenever your body decides. Nature will dictate." What I mean is that once we have regained control of our eating patterns based on our real hunger, eating only when we need to rather than when custom or pressure dictates, our bodies settle into a natural rhythm and remain at a steady, healthy weight for our height, age and shape.

We can all reach this state once we realize that the way we eat and drink is entirely up to us. Our past, our environment and our way of life may well influence it, but food is not the issue. It's the result. For example, when I had a weight problem, almost every morning I would enjoy a croissant with my coffee as I had done for most of my life. Once I lost touch with my hunger, I'd sometimes consume three croissants for breakfast before I'd even finished my first coffee. I don't deny myself that pleasure now by any means, but instead I'll enjoy a single croissant slowly, taking the time to really savour it and giving my body the time it needs to let me know when I'm full.

When we analyse the triggers that affect our eating habits with a loving self-awareness, rather than with the obsessive control that so often dominates our thinking when it comes to food, and if we become more mindful of the issues that subconsciously challenge us, then we can learn to control our weight in ways we've never experienced before.

With my help, all these things are possible if we work together to unlock these inner secrets in a safe and caring way. By following my guidelines, I can help you on the path to achieving the weight you want to be and set your mind and body free.

What is psychotherapy?

According to the American Psychological Association, psychotherapy is "a collaborative treatment" between an individual and a therapist where the latter uses "scientifically validated procedures to help people develop healthier, more effective habits". It often takes the form of four steps – connecting with the client and understanding their pain; exploring their issues further; explaining how those issues may have come about; and teaching them coping skills. It is a nurturing, supportive experience in which trust is established early on and the therapist/client relationship becomes a way of working together to identify unhealthy negative behaviours and replace them with healthy, positive ones.

Drawn from my own experience as a psychotherapist and case studies from the hundreds of clients I've helped and continue to help, this book will give you simple tools you can use to distinguish between the messages your body sends you when it's hungry from those sent by your emotions.

You will find a Food and Emotions Diary that will be discussed at length as well as a week's worth of blank diary pages at the end of the book.

Use them. Write in them. Make them yours.

Also at the back of this book are some blank Notes pages that you can use to write down your answers to the questions you're going to be asking yourself.

Keep both your Diary and Notes pages as a handy guide. Look at them frequently. Remind yourself how far you have come as you progress through the changes I will help you make.

Be brave.
Surprise yourself.

Change can take time but with a few psychological strategies to incorporate into your daily life, I promise I can help you on the path to self-revelation, setting both your body and your mind free. I know this because it has not only worked for so many others – it also worked for me.

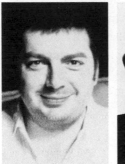 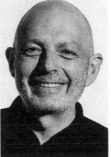

1

HOW MUCH WOULD YOU LIKE TO WEIGH?

"I wish I was as skinny as when I first met my husband. Back then, we used to wear the same size jeans. Even then, I felt overweight. I only wish now that I was as thin as I was when I thought I was fat."

Whenever a new client walks into my therapy room wanting to lose weight, especially if they seem happy and successful, I know instinctively that they have a secret.

Something has happened in their lives that has impacted them in some way, has had a direct effect on their self-perception and especially on their relationship with food. I only have to scratch the surface to find out what that is and then it becomes my role to try to help them deal with those issues.

The majority of my clients come to me primarily because they don't like their body the way it is. They think that if they can just get slim then everything else in their lives will change for the better. They might be hungry to find the man or woman of their dreams, or long to rekindle their flagging sex lives. They may believe that being thinner will make them more popular, allow them to achieve the success they seek, or help them win the award they've been nominated for.

Plagued by low self-worth, they call themselves greedy or worse – "fat cow" is probably the most common expression I hear from those who tell me they feel doomed to live the rest of their lives with their "unattractive" body after repeated efforts to lose weight have failed.

Even though they instinctively know that if they eat less, exercise more, avoid processed foods and cut down on alcohol, the weight will not only fall off but also stay off, they no longer trust themselves to make those kinds of decisions. No matter how educated and intelligent they are, they often seem to have lost all common sense and come to me seeking a manual of what, how and when to eat.

Several anxiously ask me, "Will I ever be able to eat potatoes again?" or, "Do you think I should take turmeric supplements?" or, "Is it five or ten pieces of fruit and vegetables that I should eat every day?"

The truth is they usually know as much about healthy eating as I do. Desperate for answers, they've become amateur experts on the subject, reading all the articles they can find, buying every new "clean eating" cookbook, watching all the diet television programmes, and attending all sorts of classes and seminars.

When I tell them that I'm not the oracle and that I don't issue conventional diet sheets, I can sense both their incredulity and their disappointment. "No foods are taboo," I explain. "Besides, you already know what's healthy and what you should and shouldn't be eating. You just need to find the balance that's right for you."

One of the first questions I ask any new client is, "How much would you like to weigh?" It doesn't matter to me if their answer is eight or fifteen stone, fifty or a hundred kilos, or whether they talk in dress or waist sizes rather than pounds. What I'm more interested in is the answer to my next question, "And when were you last that weight?"

Their response almost always relates to a time in their lives when they were happiest with their bodies – such as the bride who lost a lot of weight before her wedding day and "never looked better", or the stock market trader who used to go running every morning before work at a time when his job and his life "still excited" him.

The image they have in their minds of the slimmer, younger person they once were can often take on a romantic, nostalgic quality that probably can't now be matched realistically. A 55-year-old mother of three is never going to look as she did when she was 19, and a 60-something man with arthritic knees is unlikely to be as fit as he was when he was 21, no matter how much weight he loses. By setting themselves unachievable goals, they are already sabotaging their attempts to achieve their dream weight in a way they may not consciously appreciate.

Some people answer differently. For example, they might be morbidly obese and only want to lose a few stones or kilos when – for health reasons alone – they could easily lose a lot more.

"When were you last that weight?" I ask again, and although they might recount some moment when they felt happiest with their bodies, I realize that they've set themselves a low target chiefly because they are scared of raising their expectations too high.

> **"I feel so fat and ugly I can hardly stand to look at myself in the mirror. No wonder my partner doesn't want anything to do with me in bed. I can't believe how much I've let myself go."**

Many who seek my help aren't seriously overweight at all but have convinced themselves that they are. They constantly check their own bodies and grimace at themselves in the mirror before driving themselves and their families crazy with all the things they feel obliged to do to reach their "perfect" weight.

Some of their techniques can be extreme, like those who frequently have colonic irrigation or exist on a carb-free, gluten-free, alkaline-only diet. I know a few who live exclusively on raw meat in the hope that they'll pick up a tapeworm.

One woman told me in all seriousness, "I sleep naked with no duvet and the window wide open so that my core temperature plummets and I lose weight overnight." It was the depths of winter and I'd already noticed that she was only wearing a T-shirt and jeans.

"But what about your husband?" I asked gently.

"Oh, he sleeps in the spare room."

Then there are those who have spent thousands of pounds on fad diets – anything from hi-tech juicers to vile green gunk – and have been led to believe that all these things will have lasting effects. They think nothing of placing their entire families on a similarly radical regime in order not to even handle tempting foods. "I haven't eaten bread in five years. I won't even allow it into the house."

Perversely, mothers frequently tell me how worried they are about the legacy they're passing on to their children by their compulsive, obsessive behaviour. "How can I prevent my kids from becoming as fixated on their weight as I've always been?" they plead.

Some voluntarily undergo invasive surgery such as stomach stapling or the insertion of inflatable balloons to physically prevent them from overeating. They know this is a potentially risky procedure, yet even then many find tricks to cheat the surgery such as overeating ice cream or drinking lots of sugary drinks just to feel full.

What they don't expect are the emotional consequences that occur once such radical measures begin to produce results, even with their cheating. Unless they are psychologically prepared to drop so much weight so quickly, then these kinds of surgical patients can often find themselves suffering from depression. If food was their only comfort and they have lost the pleasure of enjoying it, then they suddenly feel horribly exposed and all alone. They didn't have enough lead-in time to change their eating habits and way of thinking before it was suddenly imposed on them.

On several occasions I've been shocked to hear clients openly confess to me their wish that they might develop cancer so that they can lose some weight. "Just a minor type," they add hastily, reading my expression. "Something I could recover from following treatment – after I've got down to the size I want."

What they are losing isn't weight but all sense of reason in their pursuit of what they've been brainwashed into thinking is the ideal body. The amount of weight they want to lose doesn't matter. Sometimes losing one or two kilos (three or four pounds) can be much more painful and difficult than losing a great deal more, and can take longer. It all depends where the problem is rooted.

> **"I never feel like I show people the real me. I am putting on a front for those around me – my husband, my children and my colleagues. Inside, I'm full of anxiety and fear and that's what keeps driving me back to food."**

Most of the men, women and teenagers who come to see me already have a very clear idea in their minds of their target weight, which often relates to dropping a few sizes or achieving a healthy Body Mass Index (see page 34).

They may have a specific event they want to slim down for, such as a wedding, a school reunion, a holiday or a significant birthday. If that is the case, I need to make sure that they don't subconsciously plan to put all the weight back on afterward, as the event itself should not be their only goal.

What they really want – whether they realize it or not – is to be free from all the anxiety surrounding their excess weight. They are carrying so much on their shoulders that they can't even think straight. The emotional weight is a far heavier burden than the physical, and very often they've been carrying it around with them for decades.

In an effort to free ourselves from the unwelcome emotional load we all carry, it's important to build up a clear picture of our eating patterns, by noticing when and what we eat. Later, you'll start filling in the daily Food and Emotions Diary I mentioned in the Introduction, but to begin with you can think gently about your habits around food. Let's start by asking yourself the following three questions:

- **Do you eat quickly or slowly?** This is one of the most important questions I ask. Most people with weight issues eat too fast, and I have rarely come across a slow eater who's overweight. This is because the more slowly we eat the more time we give our brain to receive and process the messages from our body that it has had enough.

- **How hungry are you when you sit down to eat?** The answer will obviously vary but it's a question we can all ask ourselves, especially when we are preparing quantities of food at home, or are in a restaurant considering a menu. Are we truly in need of food or just gearing up to eat because this is the allotted time, or because someone expects us to?

- **Do you really feel hungry enough to eat a three-course meal?** Maybe you need only a starter or a main? Why not try a smaller portion eaten slowly and see how full you are before choosing to cook or order anything else? It's possible that this will be enough, or that you only want to add a small side dish.

These issues are the kinds I work on a lot and we will come back to them later, because so many people have completely lost touch with their perception of hunger and eat too quickly, only out of habit, to comfort themselves or to please someone else. Some might say, "A colleague in the office was handing out slices of her birthday cake so even though I'd just finished my sandwich I still had some as it looked so good and I didn't want to appear rude."

Another client might tell me, "My partner cooks me dinner after a busy day every night so I feel it's the least I can do to eat it even if I'm not that hungry."

A third might confess, "Six of us went out for Chinese food as usual and got overexcited and over-ordered. I ended up trying a bit of everything on the table until I was so full I could hardly stand up."

My intention is to make you fully aware of the triggers that surround us all and, more importantly, teach you how to handle them. If we learn to understand what's making us feel hungry in the first place, then we can recognize when we are most vulnerable to temptation, and why. I call it the Hunger Game.

Instead of feeling guilty each time we eat, we have to learn to take some responsibility for our own actions. For many of us our way of life is hectic and we eat on the run, not being mindful enough about how hungry we really are and what we really feel like eating. The usual pattern that follows is to chastise ourselves for consuming more than we really needed, and immediately start complaining that we feel horribly bloated or fat.

The trick is to understand that you need to stop feeling guilty and start taking responsibility. There are reasons for what you do. No one is forcing food into your mouth.

"I gulp everything down so quickly that I usually feel the effects of my overeating immediately after a meal with acid indigestion and an uncomfortable sense of being bloated."

The way in which we take in our food is also important. The following pointers may sound simplistic to begin with, but if you keep to them each time you eat, you'll be amazed how much difference they can make to your relationship with food.

■ **Sit comfortably and in a relaxed, upright position:** not standing up at a takeaway counter, perched on the arm of a chair, or hunched over the plate ready to shovel food in. Many of us literally lean into our plates, keeping our heads down, and wolfing down food as a way of avoidance or because we're stressed about how little time we have. We might not want to engage with those around us because they're difficult or annoying. We may eat solidly so as not to be interrupted and to avoid eye contact.

■ **Take a few breaths before eating and between mouthfuls:** Whatever emotional baggage we bring to each meal, it's important to first take a few breaths to trigger our body's relaxation response. Whenever we take quicker, shorter breaths our body remains in a state of tension and we tend to eat even faster. We don't have to sit there inhaling and exhaling in any kind of dramatic way. It can be very discreet and takes just a few seconds.

■ **Take a moment to consider what's in front of you:** If we take a few seconds to look at our food and smell it in a mindful way, then we can really start to think about how hungry we are and what we will start with. Perhaps we're thirsty rather than hungry? Maybe try drinking some water first; we can see if that helps fill us up.

■ **Be aware of what you choose to eat first and why:** The way in which we tackle the food on our plates is interesting psychologically and may dictate the amount you have unconsciously programmed yourself to consume. Do you tend to begin with the food you like best, or do you leave it to last? Some of us systematically take a little bit of each item, afraid of missing out on a thing. Others start with what they like least, and save the best until last. This is because many of us like to have the taste of our favourite foods in our mouths at the end, without appreciating that saving the best until last is another subconscious inducement to keep going and finish the plate even if we are full. The truth is we don't have to. Try starting with the best bits and see if that makes you less inclined to finish your meal.

Eat slowly: Once we begin to eat, it helps to slow right down, being sure to taste every mouthful of food and enjoy its texture and subtleties as we chew. People eat quickly for different reasons. Some people feel so embarrassed about their weight that they don't like to be seen eating, and bolt their food to get through what is no longer a pleasurable experience. If the food on the table was something to be competed for, say, in a large family, at boarding school, or in some other situation, then we may wolf it down so quickly that we don't even know we're sated, because the ten minutes it took us to devour the meal is still ten minutes short of the moment the stomach informs the brain that we've had enough.

Try not to overeat with each mouthful: Putting a lot of food in our mouth all at once can bring a sense of almost childlike comfort and reassurance, but it isn't healthy as it can often encourage us to eat still more. Only when we breathe normally, eat less at a time, and decelerate can we digest our food properly. Reducing your intake with these simple little steps will help you on your journey to a far healthier relationship with food.

Don't anticipate your next mouthful: One of the cleverest tricks to slow down your eating is to never load up a fork for the next mouthful until you've finished the one you're eating. Doing so only speeds up the process, while the sight of the loaded fork waiting for us becomes a tantalizing psychological incentive to guzzle everything even faster. If you put down your cutlery between every mouthful, this doesn't happen. Use that short pause to look up and engage in conversation, show interest in others, read something, or watch the television. All these activities help to slow us down and take our minds off the mission to clear our plate. Eating doesn't have to be a race to the finish every time, so try to linger and you'll be surprised how much more you enjoy the experience.

- **Reassess your hunger throughout each meal:** Only by taking regular pauses can we re-evaluate how hungry we are, asking ourselves throughout the meal, "Am I still enjoying this? Have I had enough now?" Only if the answer is yes can you commit to fully enjoying the experience. Once we are no longer hungry, we don't enjoy our food nearly as much, so by changing things in this way we can experiment with our hunger and see what helps us to eat less.

- **Stop when you are full:** There is a very common compulsion to finish everything on our plates. If our parents grew up in troubled times, as mine did, then it might have been drummed into us from an early age to always eat everything on our plate, even if we are full. Accept that you don't have to. Two justifications are frequently mentioned when it comes to understanding this diktat. First, it would be rude not to eat the entire contents of the plate that your host has presented to you. They have gone to the trouble of cooking, and they expect you to do them the honour of eating everything they have served. You also give them the recognition they expect from you. And if in addition they prepared the food with love, how dare you refuse part of that love? The second justification is something most of us heard our parents tell us from childhood – "There are children dying of starvation in Africa." It is true that we live in a world where many people are hungry and sometimes die from starvation, so it seems criminal and arrogant to think of throwing food away rather than eating it. But if you think about it, eating when your body tells you it has had enough is twice the waste: for the planet and for your health.

Habits often seem hard to change, and this can take time. We've usually been eating in the same pattern for years, and we have to be gentle with ourselves if we want to achieve these changes. The thing to remember is that our body knows when we have had enough, and it lets us know. It is truly one of the finest mechanisms on earth. We ignore it at our peril, because it will only store the excess calories as fat, adding layer upon layer until we finally realize that we need to stop.

The good thing is that we'll see the benefits of a change in our habits quite quickly: our meals will tend to be less stressful, we'll feel better about ourselves, we'll have more energy for other things and then, yes, we'll lose weight.

"It wasn't until I started to really think about how and when I ate that I realized I was going through the motions most of the time. It was as if I was on automatic pilot – like some mindless machine munching its way through the day."

There is a thin line between mindfulness and control. Some people eagerly tell me, "Oh, the things you told me have already made a huge difference to how I eat, Philippe. I'm really going to watch myself from now on."

This isn't what I mean by mindful awareness. It's vital not to obsess, but to try to make it more of a game. We need to listen to ourselves instead of watching ourselves. Then we can think gently and with self-kindness about how we eat, becoming much more aware of the signals our body is sending us, and make more careful decisions about the food on our plates.

This needn't be done in a way that adds to any existing fixation, but in a way that allows us to rediscover food sensations and take our time deciding exactly what we want next. This allows our brain to let us know what it really needs, how much, and when.

All of these strategies are simple but effective ways of allowing us to achieve the weight we desire and become the author of our life's next chapter. They also teach us to be kinder to ourselves. This is very important because almost all of my clients tell me they are unhappy, and I note that they are impossibly hard on themselves, with a terrible self-image.

"I'm such a pig!" they frequently cry.

"That's strange, because you don't look like a pig and you don't smell like one either," I reply with a smile. "You have a good career, you've successfully raised your children, you dress well, you're smart, and your friends and family love you. Why are you so down on yourself?"

In therapy, this kind of praise often sparks tears as people become extremely emotional about their problems and insecurities, especially once they start to believe that things could be different. This is because our self-perception about who we are and what we look like is often shaped by how stressed we feel, or how put upon. And so many of us go through life feeling that we are taking care of everyone else's needs but not our own. We are hungry for more "me" time. We've come to accept that life isn't fair and we are just trying to do the best we can and find our way. We long to unburden ourselves of all the difficult emotions we may have been harbouring for years – inner feelings that only we know about (our secrets) – and from which we can often seek distraction and comfort in food and alcohol.

Most of all we want to respect and love ourselves.

Change is scary. For some people it's too frightening to deal with, but I know from facing my own demons that the rewards are truly worth the effort.

> **"I've struggled with diet after diet my whole life and have always failed. I never thought I'd succeed. Since I've lost the weight I feel almost evangelical about it. I want everyone to know that there is a way to do it."**

Ask yourself the following questions without judgment or disapproval, but in a way that's benevolent and loving. Be kind to yourself, and remember this is just a way of getting you to start thinking about your eating habits and the way you regard yourself.

Write down your answers honestly, then take the time to really think about them and to acknowledge the way in which you consume food and why. Look at these questions and answers frequently, building up a self-awareness that will allow you to see yourself in a gentle, non-judgmental way.

How much would you like to weigh, or what size would you like to be?

If you are unsure what weight is healthy for you, then a good tool to use is the Body Mass Index, or BMI. You can calculate this online via a number of websites (see page 265 for my recommendations). Most BMI calculators ask you to enter your gender, age, height and weight, plus an indication of how active you are. The tool then gives you a number that comes up on a scale somewhere between underweight and obese, showing the healthy range for your size. It might also suggest a recommended daily calorie intake and tell you how much you can try to lose to put you in the middle of the healthier range.

Once you have this information, you can compare it to the weight you wanted to be in your mind and decide if that now seems realistic. If it is too low or too high, ask yourself how you came up with that number. A target weight that is lower than recommended for a healthy BMI will probably leave you with a feeling of failure if you can't achieve it. Most importantly of all, it could be dangerous physically if you do.

Some may opt for a number less than the ideal weight as a safety measure – "just in case I put a bit of weight back on." Psychologically, this gives us permission to keep playing with our weight within the range we've selected, but the downside is that it can lead to a yo-yo effect with the constant gaining or losing of a few pounds, which will tend to become bigger with time. Before even starting to lose weight we have over-analysed the process in a toxic way, setting ourselves up for disappointment.

A target weight that is higher than recommended for a healthy BMI shouldn't be regarded as showing a lack of ambition or commitment. It usually reflects the fears we might have, and these deserve to be taken seriously too. What do these fears tell us? That eating healthily will take too much time; that we will never get below that number; that losing too much weight might affect your relationships with others ...? Clients often complain, "But I'll have to change all my clothes," or, "I'll be too sexy and won't know how to handle seduction," or, "Other people might start to envy me."

It is important to address these fears and see if they really make sense in your life today. Is the risk of changing and moving out of your comfort zone bigger than the risk of staying within it? Losing weight will take time and happen gradually, so take another look at these fears at the different stages of your weight loss. As your weight goes down, your confidence will grow and your views on how you feel and how other people think of you will change.

Another good exercise is to write down any fears you have at the beginning and put them away in a drawer, or perhaps a mental briefcase. Every now and again throughout this process, open that drawer or briefcase and take a look at them again to see if they are still as valid. You may be surprised by the answer.

When were you last your ideal weight, and is your goal realistic?

If your target weight is the same as the weight you were when you were exercising frequently and this is something you won't be able to do regularly, you should set your weight higher if you want it to be sustainable. The same applies if your general way of life has become much more sedentary because of your age or time constraints, or for health reasons. You can, of course, decide to take positive steps to change that, but we'll get to the subject of exercise later on.

It is also very common for people to choose their target weight or desired dress or waist size based on something they've read or seen in the media. This is especially true for young people addicted to social media, but it also applies to adults who tell me how they feel influenced by people they see in magazines who have recently lost weight. If we identify with a celebrity because of some slight physical resemblance, or see someone on the television that's in the kind of shape we'd like to be in, then it is natural to aspire to that. We can also often relate to someone we know and admire – a relative perhaps, or a best friend, someone we work with, even a fellow passenger on a commuter train.

What you have to remember is that we are all very different, and in many ways – our height, age, way of life, tastes, metabolism, genetics, family history. Your healthy weight will (and can only) reflect who you are. It cannot be achieved by trying to fit into a group or body type that you don't belong to. This is your body, your story and your way of life. Whatever you decide to do to change, it needs to reflect on you and you alone – not on people you may know or wish you could be like.

It isn't healthy to compare yourself with people who are really slim or fit, even though this may be very difficult for some people to accept. You can make the necessary changes, but it is up to you to set clear and realistic goals.

When did things change with your body shape, and why?

Most of my clients seek my help after years of struggling with their weight. When I ask them how long they've been unhappy about their body image they very often respond, "As far back as I can remember." Shockingly, many can't recall one moment in their life when they were happy with how they looked. They either had no experience of it or they'd forgotten about it, and this is also true of people who have only recently started to gain weight.

I ask them, "Were you still unhappy with your body when you were, say, 18, or maybe 25?" The answer is still usually yes.

If this is true for you too, then try looking back at some old photographs of yourself at those ages and ask yourself how they make you feel now. More often than not, I hear people tell me that, although they weren't happy with themselves back then, they would be more than happy with that body shape now.

"Look at me! I thought I was so fat, but I wasn't fat at all! I would love to have a body like that now."

This revelation often makes them sad for the young person that they once were, and how they struggled with their unhappiness for no real reason. "How could I have been so self-critical so young? I wasn't overweight at all!" The benefit of hindsight gives them a more distanced perception of events and emotions they may have felt in the past – feelings that might well have been triggered by their parents or others making random comments about their weight or their diet in a way that made them unhappy and self-conscious.

By proving to ourselves that there was a time when we could and should have been happy with our bodies but still weren't, we can come to a dawning realization that it really didn't have much to do with the size and shape we were but with our own insecurities or lack of self-confidence. Once we accept this, we can address that as the issue that underlies the way we feel now about how we look, then use the understanding we have gained in order not to pursue an unachievable goal for our current plans.

In my therapy, I often use Transactional Analysis, according to which we each have three separate ego states in a constant state of dialogue: the Child, the Parent and the Adult (see opposite). These three states of the "self" coexist in all of us and express themselves independently according to the circumstances. They define not only our relationship to others, but to ourselves as well.

Almost every day I hear my clients start a sentence with, "I know it's silly, but . . ." judging themselves before they even tell me what they want to say. They subconsciously want to put me in the Parent position during our sessions, which will automatically place them in the Child ego state, as this is something they have not only become accustomed to but also absolves them of responsibility. It is my role to help them understand that by constantly expecting others to judge them in this way, or by judging themselves, they are not fully owning their feelings or their actions.

I'll talk about this a bit more later, but by understanding how these ego states are constantly chattering to each other in our minds, we can start to bring the Adult into many of our own situations to help us see that our unhappiness about our lives or how we look is in our own hands.

Transactional Analysis

Transactional Analysis is a method of therapy used by psychotherapists. It is based on the principle that our behaviour, especially our communication within social relationships, is an interaction with our surroundings according to the three facets of our personality – the Child, the Parent and the Adult. The Child is spontaneous, dependent, but also creative and intuitive. It represents the feelings of life, according to various sensations and motivations. The Parent can be nurturing but also overcritical. It often manifests as moral judgments and protective attitudes. The Adult is usually logical and rational. It inquires, assesses, analyses and decides. Each of these ego states is vital for our normal development and growth, and should be in balance in a healthy way. When the balance goes awry and one facet becomes more dominant than the others, Transactional Analysis diagnoses how much of the "me" intervenes in relationships and allows the individual to harness all three aspects appropriately to regain control.

The truth is that various things happen in our lives that can impact our behaviour. Overeating and drinking too much is a simplistic way of coping with difficult times and the emotions we don't know how to manage properly.

It doesn't even have to be a major trauma like the loss of a parent or a job – it can sometimes be events that others might handle easily but which seem more difficult for us. It could be the waning of a sex life or a competitive situation at work. It can be something as simple as an off-the-cuff remark.

In order to be more aware of the emotions we're dealing with from the past, we need to do some introspection. This is the point at which it is worthwhile to pinpoint the event or series of events that triggered a change in your food consumption and/or your weight gain.

When did you first start self-medicating with food and/or alcohol?

For many women, it was marriage and then pregnancy that was the catalyst for change. For men, it can often be marriage and fatherhood. For younger people, the adolescent years can herald the start of a dramatic change in eating habits, for good or bad.

Whatever the trigger, recognizing it can be scary, especially if you are opening up old wounds that you've hidden from everyone including yourself. We'll discuss this more later. The trick is to realize exactly when the change occurred and to try to remember the person you were back then, compared to the person you are now. Were you happier, less stressed? Did you have more exciting prospects ahead in your life?

What is the secret that may be affecting your self-worth?

We build self-confidence at a very young age and the way our parents or adult relatives react to us when we're children can be decisive. Too many parents tend to label children in all kinds of different ways and this label can stick with us our whole life, unless we come to realize it at some point.

For example, a mother might tell her friends, "My son Andrew is so lazy. All he cares about is food," and these labels will lodge in Andrew's brain. I often hear parents declare that their child is going to be an artist, and I want to tell them, "Don't say that. They might end up being a scientist or a mechanic." These kinds of projections can have an enormous impact on young and pliable minds.

My mother used to tell me when I was a teenager that I was like a nomad travelling from place to place with a suitcase, and in many ways that is what I have become, perhaps because I heard it from her so many times. Our life story is often written by others and we can grow up thinking, "Okay, this is who I am and this is how my life will be."

We can refer to this as our "life script", which is often not a conscious path but can still secretly dictate many of the decisions we make and the beliefs we have about who we are. If our parents were hypercritical about how we looked, ate or behaved, or if they put us on a diet when we were young, this can affect our own self-image enormously. If we had parents who were obsessed about the way they looked, or compared us unfavourably with our siblings or their friends' children, then this can also make us unhappy.

We all have this kind of secret scenario in our heads, and we often have a sense of guilt if we do not fulfil the wishes or live up to the expectations of our parents – whether they are dead or alive. The good news is that this doesn't have to shape us. We each have the right to be different, to have fun, to experience different things, to maybe not get married and have kids, or not be a university lecturer, or an artist.

The choice is ours.

TO RECAP

- Be kinder to yourself, more accepting and forgiving – all of us have secrets that affect our self-worth.

- Find the balance that is right for you – we all know what is healthy and what we should be doing. This won't happen straight away but will evolve naturally.

- Be realistic about your target weight.

- Connect with your hunger and listen to your body signals.

- Slow down and pay attention to everything from your posture to your decision to keep eating.

- Tune into your own emotions, past and present, and see what they are telling you about your past, present and future.

- Be in the Adult ego state when reflecting on your patterns, instead of judging them through the prism of your Parent.

CASE STUDY

Sue is a 46-old mother of two grown-up children, who are both away studying at university. I use the word "mother" intentionally, as this is how Sue describes herself.

In a previous life she was a successful publicist, until she got pregnant. As a child, Sue had missed her mother, who was often busy, and she didn't want her children to experience that, so she and her husband decided it would make sense for her to quit her job. That's when she stopped seeing herself as a "woman" and became a full-time carer.

By taking on this domestic, maternal role, however, Sue felt unable to do anything about the weight she'd gained during her two pregnancies, or stop herself from adding more year after year. Full of guilt, she tried six different diets but the weight always crept back on, and she continued to gain. Feeling helpless and trapped, she was caught in the classic yo-yo effect.

During our first session, it very quickly became clear that Sue was not happy with her life balance. She insisted that she needed to lose 31 kilos (5 stone) – to get back to the weight she had been when she felt most fulfilled as a young working woman. Even though she tried to keep busy, she was often bored. Food was her main source of distraction and had become a kind of comforting companion – available anywhere and anytime. She thought about food almost the entire day, whether she was on a diet or not – planning what she'd buy and cook, and thinking about what she should or shouldn't eat.

Her husband was busier than ever in a career that kept him working long hours, often away from home. It was difficult for him to understand her guilt about having a relatively easy life and her concerns and frustrations about her weight. She longed to be back to the size she was before she had children, when she was working, successful and newly married.

I helped Sue to realize that she needed to take back control of her life and rediscover the person she was before she had children. I accompanied her on this journey, showing her how she could feed herself with something other than food. When eating to excess becomes your main distraction and your chief companion, it can be very frightening to give it up unless you have something else to replace it with.

After giving it some thought, Sue joined a yoga class, which helped her reconnect to her own body. Then she came up with the idea of starting a new business with a friend.

As her mind became less focused on food and her weight, she learned how to be more mindful about eating and very quickly her portions grew much smaller and she stopped binge eating. Sue lost three and a half stone (19 kilos) in seven months and has stayed at that weight for the last four years. The loss may not have been as much as what she initially had in mind, but she was nevertheless delighted with the change in her body and in her attitude to life.

Like many people, Sue thought that being slim again would open the door to a new life but, in truth, it is by welcoming new projects into our lives that we empower ourselves to be happy with the body we have.

2

WHAT BENEFITS DO YOU GAIN FROM BEING OVERWEIGHT?

"I've been fat since I was a kid. It's just the way I am. I've always been known as the joker, the jovial boy who makes everyone laugh. If I lose all this weight, then I'm afraid that people won't like me so much. Maybe I won't like myself anymore, and that scares me."

It may sound like a bizarre question, but within the very first session I ask all my clients, "What benefits do you gain from being overweight?" They are often surprised, but the question makes perfect sense. Even though we might genuinely want to lose those extra pounds, understanding the real reasons why we struggle to do so is essential to finally escaping the cycle.

Most of us believe that we overeat because we don't have any self-discipline, or because we like food too much. "I'm so greedy that I disgust myself" is a common refrain, as is, "I have zero willpower."

This is almost never the case. It often takes just as much willpower and energy to keep the weight on as it does to take it off. In finding out what's at the heart of the issue, we can experience something of a revelation once we truly get to know ourselves.

For example, the majority of those who come to see me are women and most of them have issues with their size. Time and again I hear them say that they no longer feel sexually desirable because of the weight they've put on over the years.

They cannot grasp the concept that many people consider larger women attractive, or that their partners might still find them sexy regardless of their size because of the way they dress, think or respond to physical contact. Much depends on the way their partner behaves and if they feel they're being judged.

"So what benefits are there to you in remaining overweight?" I ask. "If it makes you feel so undesirable, do you believe your excess weight protects you from the attentions of your partner?"

You may be surprised by how many say yes.

One client confessed, "My husband knows I don't like him to see me naked or run his hands over my fat body, so as long as I stay this size we don't need to have sex."

Another told me, "My wife's jealous when other women even glance at me, so if I don't look good they don't respond and then she's not so reactive."

A man in his forties said, "I love my partner but I have a very high sex drive and if I lost weight I'd feel even sexier and want a lover younger than the one I'm with. It's safer for the status quo to remain the way I am."

Some of my clients were abused as children and feel responsible in some way, so they punish themselves by remaining overweight and thus – as they see it – staying safely unattractive. "It was partly my fault," they tell me. "Back then I used to look like I was asking for it. These days, I don't."

Some women think that if they stay "chubby" then they'll blend in more easily socially, and not be regarded as competitive by those around them, especially other females. "All the women in my office are a lot younger than me and so much skinnier, so I'm the mumsy one. They look up to me and don't regard me as a threat."

It is a sad fact of life that those around overweight people tend to feel some sort of moral superiority over them. Thinking of us as weak or unhappy, they feel sorry for us and assume we won't perform well, so they often stop asking too much of us, or – in a work situation – they give a task to someone else. For some of us, this "invisibility" and the easing of pressure that comes with it in a social or work environment can sometimes feel like another benefit.

———————

There are all kinds of other gains from carrying extra weight. Some people who are desperately lonely, either within an unhappy relationship or living alone, come to regard their overeating as a kind of slow death – a social suicide that, if unchecked, can become a physical suicide as well.

Others use it as an emotional tool, or even a weapon. A middle-aged woman who sought my help used her size as a kind of passive-aggressive revenge on her unfaithful husband, expressing her anger by gaining weight in response to both his inappropriate behaviour and his frequently unkind remarks. Another woman who feared she was losing her looks deployed her weight as a kind of test to see if she was loved for who she really was, not for what she looked like.

People often allow their weight to define them and then they create a persona to match their appearance. An opera singer who became a client was afraid that if she lost the 25 kilos (4 stone) she wanted, she'd lose the power and strength of her voice. A comedian who came to see me believed people wouldn't think he was as funny anymore if he was slender. An actress felt much the same, worried that she wouldn't get the same kind of "jolly" roles. They were all proven wrong in the end and acknowledged that they had partly used their persona as an excuse.

> **"Each time I binged it felt like I was literally squashing all my unhappy thoughts down inside me for a while. It felt good to eat. It comforted me. When I was eating I felt safe because I didn't have to think."**

Perhaps the most common benefit from overeating, though, is the way it masks our inner unhappiness and puts our unwanted emotions to sleep.

"Comfort" and "security" are key words when it comes to food. From our first day on this earth, we are taught to understand that food is both nourishment and love. If someone is feeding us then that means they're caring for us and making sure we don't starve or get dehydrated.

Food means we are not alone.

Food is love.

By the time we have reached adulthood we have spent our lives being nurtured and comforted by food, which also has a physical and biological effect on the way our bodies and minds feel, releasing mood-enhancing chemicals in a way that little else can. So if we relinquish the comfort that overeating brings us, what do we have to put in its place?

"I've spent most of my life being afraid," one client admitted to me during a session. "If I give up the relief that eating food gives me, I'm even more afraid that I'll have to confront all those fears without any kind of safety net."

Many people believe that if they could only lose weight they'd be happy, but they also secretly fear that being slim won't bring them the joy they seek. If it doesn't, then this will expose the fact that they are unhappy for other reasons, so they decide it is better to stay the way they are and not risk the disappointment.

The truth is that the less we need comfort because our lives are comforting enough, the less we will need comfort food.

The three main emotions that we usually try to quash by overeating are anger, fear and sadness. We can carry some of these around with us for years. They may relate to a trauma we've suffered in our childhood or a difficult experience we've been through at some other point in our life.

These aren't always negative emotions, though. They are each a valid expression of our feelings and can be worked on to our advantage. We need to acknowledge them, accept them and understand how to use them for the greater good. If we don't express these important emotions, they can fester and deepen to create a toxic cycle.

Our anger can be harnessed to set limits and boundaries and help change things that we find unacceptable. Once we recognize what we are angry about and why, we can turn our anger back, positively and non-aggressively, on the people who made us feel that way. Our fear is an important part of our psyche and one that helps us survive, but it can easily take over. By removing ourselves from that which makes us fearful, either by turning off bad news or allowing ourselves the space to relax, dream and breathe, we can switch off from the fear and regain our inner balance.

Our sadness is something we often feel ashamed of and try to hide; yet it is as valid as all our other emotions and needs to be expressed in a controlled, safe environment to release the tension and permit ourselves to feel.

It may not be easy to figure out which of these emotions we're feeling when we're eating more than we need – or even when we're not eating, as these feelings are ever-present whether we're conscious of them or not.

Becoming more aware and understanding what is preoccupying our minds allows us to eat more mindfully. We can't fully focus on the physical sensations and other messages that our body is sending us if we're absorbed or even overwhelmed by something else.

"I never had a problem with my eating until I was stuck at home with the kids. I chose to be a house husband and it was great, but I did become resentful when most of my days revolved around their needs and there was never any time for mine."

These secret emotions we all have inside us only add to what I call our daily emotional load: the bundle of feelings that we're constantly burdened with. This load can be increased by so many different things – what we see in the press, a conversation we're having or hearing, our relationship with others, work or personal issues. We can be upset by the attitude of someone or moved by a sound, a smell or a memory.

Our brains are never at rest, and we collect and collate hundreds of thousands of pieces of information every hour – many of which have a direct effect on our emotions. This can be conscious, for example if we hear some sad news about someone we like, or more subconscious, such as the aroma of a favourite perfume, or the smile on a stranger's face.

None of these emotions is "bad", but at some point they might overwhelm our minds and this can make us act and eat inappropriately. Once we notice our behaviour, it's usually too late and we start feeling bad and often guilty about our response.

It isn't always easy to figure out which feelings we're dealing with, so a good trick is to find out what we're thinking about at the specific moment we begin to eat. This will usually enable us to find out which emotions or mix of emotions have been triggered.

For example, let's say we're thinking about a holiday to France we're planning next summer. We might be telling ourselves:

- I'm really looking forward to relaxing. (happiness)

- Can I really afford it? (anxiety)

- I didn't even want to go to France. Why wasn't I more assertive? (anger)

- It will feel strange to return to the place I visited with my late father. (sadness)

This process of reflection takes only a few seconds but it allows us to have a clearer understanding about what we are feeling and why.

This, in turn, enables us to treat our emotions with consideration and respect rather than quashing them, or they will only add to our daily load:

- Unless we listen to our anger, we will not change the things we are angry about.

- When we don't pay attention to our fear, we can end up putting ourselves in danger.

- If we ignore our sadness, we find it difficult to move on to new experiences.

Only when we acknowledge our right to be happy can we fully enjoy happiness, so let's examine these emotions more closely and see what lies beneath each of them.

ANGER

"So much of the time, I feel like I'm bubbling over with anger. I've started to grind my teeth and bite my nails. I can't sleep at night for being cross with everyone, and I fly off the handle at the slightest thing."

Most of us don't know how to express our anger anymore, because it is almost always seen as a negative emotion. Yet anger can be a ticking time bomb inside us if not properly addressed.

From the moment we have our first infant tantrum, we're encouraged not to vent our frustration and fury. Angry children are frequently pacified with a dummy, food or sweets, told to "sit on the naughty step", or sent to their room. Sometimes they are treated with drugs – anything to calm or crush the emotions. Rarely does an adult say, "It's okay. I understand. You are justified in being angry or frustrated. Go ahead. Let it out."

As children, we might be able to get away with shouting, throwing things or breaking our toys, but once we reach adulthood we're expected to manage our emotions in a far more responsible way. Being aggressive or physical isn't allowed in today's society. God forbid we offend anyone in this politically correct world. And many of us are afraid that we'll be unable to manage our anger if we start to express it and that we'll explode.

The whole point of anger, though, is to harness it in order to manage our relationships with others and implement real change. If we get angry about something that offends us, then we can use it to help change things and ensure it doesn't happen again. It's about finding a voice and being able to say in a non-aggressive way, "No, I don't agree with that," or, "I don't like what you said," or, "I disagree with the way you did that."

We need to know and set limits and boundaries so that these kinds of situations don't arise again. If we can't express our anger then it only gets buried inside, and that can lead to overeating. It takes courage to tell someone, "Stop driving so fast. You're making me nervous," or, "Please knock before you enter," or, "Kindly let me know in future if you're going to be late."

In French there is an expression, *énoncer n'est pas dénoncer*, which means that to enunciate or voice your concerns isn't to denounce or to criticize. Just because I might express the view that I'm not happy that someone is always late doesn't mean I'm not happy with them or with our relationship, just that one aspect of it.

Many women find it easier than men to cry, and some will burst into tears rather than express themselves or confront someone to let them know they're not happy. Men, on the other hand, usually can't cry so easily and often see tears as a sign of weakness. More typically, they will express their sadness with anger, which can sometimes seem like a wholly inappropriate response. So in answer to the question, "What's going on? What's wrong?" they might respond by shouting, "Nothing! I'm all right! Leave me alone!"

We call this *une émotion racket* in French – a false or faux emotion. This is a distorted feeling that isn't authentic but which we might use in response to the triggers provided by those around us. If we do this often enough, we can numb ourselves to the authentic emotion too.

The trick is to understand that it is okay to feel angry, scared or sad. All of these emotions have a valid purpose in our lives, one of which is problem solving. Once we accept that the people who love us won't run a mile just because we open up about our true feelings, then we can relax into those feelings and allow ourselves to experience our emotions genuinely without needing to hide the truth.

"My wife calls me a grumpy old man, but she's wrong. I've been grumpy my whole life. Much of it dates back to when I lost my father as a young man. Since then I feel like I've been festering about everything, all the time."

It is so important to tell others what our limits are because many people simply don't know. And it's equally important to ask ourselves how or why we have got ourselves into a situation where we have become angry. What were we feeling? What are we willing to accept? If we don't know, then we can't begin to make it clear to others that our space has been invaded, or our time, or our bodies. I often hear clients complain, "She should have known I wouldn't be happy with this!" or, "How could he not realize that it was wrong?" Please stop assuming that others can guess what your limits are. People aren't psychic. Once you know the limits, then make sure you let others know. You may be afraid to appear pedantic or boring, but in fact stating these kinds of things once or twice will make you someone who is easier to live with because everyone knows where you stand.

Unless we express our genuine emotions at work or in social situations, we can go home still feeling this anger inside us, so we use food or drugs or alcohol as a kind of anaesthetic. It will make us feel better for a short while, but then we get angry with ourselves at what we've done and express that by turning the anger on ourselves:

"Oh no, I did it again!"
"I'm so pathetic."
"I'll never lose weight."
"I might as well finish off this bottle of wine/bag of snacks/packet of cookies."

This is such a common cycle: Anger. Eating. Guilt. Self-Loathing. Repeat.

In some instances, when we are in the company of others who are angry, we feel that we can't easily express our own anger and frustration for fear that it might spark a fresh argument. This can make us feel a new sense of isolation and of being misunderstood. Very often, people can bring this built-up aggression home and turn it against their partner, their children or their dog – those who haven't done anything to justify it. People are so afraid of confrontation that it's easier for them to express their anger to those around them than it is to those they don't know well.

So many of my clients are overwhelmed by frustration and anger, and feel that they cannot find the right ways to express these feelings. This may be old anger from their childhood – perhaps one of their parents treated them unfairly or favoured a sibling, or maybe they felt betrayed or used by someone years ago.

Sometimes we carry that deep kind of anger all our lives and this can make us an angry person for old reasons, not new ones. Each time something fresh irritates us, it's like scratching at a wound and reopening all that hurt. Unless we understand where the hurt is coming from and why we feel guilty and then eat, the toxic cycle goes on.

We can be angry with people who are long dead or no longer around to complain to, so that the emotion feels unresolved. Keeping hold of anger at a dead or absent person like this is one way of keeping the relationship alive. We can't let go.

What is helpful here is to voice our anger in a letter or to say it out loud so that we can finally release it. Doing this can be scary and sometimes overwhelming, so it isn't an easy process, especially if the person is still alive. In that instance we should write the letter but not send it, all the while making it clear exactly what the person did that upset us. Seeing it written down on paper in black and white can make it feel real. It can make us feel heard.

In wider society too, many people don't believe they are respected or heard. They feel abandoned and yet they are unable to express their anger through a lack of experience, or confidence, or the sense that they aren't allowed to.

All of us sometimes fear that if we express our anger we might end up having an argument. We're so afraid of not being able to manage anger properly that we often refrain from expressing our frustration at all. Everyone is frightened they will upset the status quo, so it's often easier to swallow that anger with the help of food or drink or drugs, which only keeps the emotions festering within.

If we do this, we will only make things worse. Our voice and our opinion has as much value as anyone else's, and we should be allowed to express ourselves in an adult way. The more we experiment with doing so, the more confidence we will gain that things can be different and that we can be heard.

FEAR

"Every day I wake up frightened of what new stresses the day will bring. Will I be treated fairly at work, or will someone be mean? How safe is it to travel on the trains, or should I take the bus? Can I afford to pay my bills this month?"

We live in a world full of fear. Quite apart from health scares, money worries, career stresses and general fears about the future, we're bombarded with horrifying global news of war and violent acts of terrorism. It is hard to know how not to be fearful.

Fear is there to protect us, however. If we smell burning, for example, then our bodies release adrenaline, which allows us to move quickly and escape from the fire. If we hear a noise in the night, then fear will help us jump out of bed and respond accordingly.

The trouble is that there are so many reasons to be fearful these days that we are in fear overload much of the time. This can make us want to hide under the duvet rather than act, ignoring the signals that are warning us that something is potentially dangerous or harmful.

Eating and drinking is a quick way to soothe these fears and make us feel more relaxed about all the things that are stressing us out. But by doing so, we are just avoiding ways to express our true emotions.

After a difficult day at work or an argument with the boss that could end up costing us our job, we tend to come home and pour ourselves a drink before eating something unhealthy like pizza or a takeaway – anything to relax and unwind. Doing this gives us a way to breathe. The trouble is, the things we are eating and drinking only put our fears to sleep for a short time. Before too long they will rise up to engulf us again.

First and foremost, we need to acknowledge and own all these emotions in a healthy, non-critical way. Only once we understand what's causing us to feel fearful, angry or sad can we take steps to do something about it and change the situation, rather than repeatedly responding in a poor or inappropriate way.

So, for example, if we find it too difficult to respond to a situation immediately, we can react later. Having given our response due thought, at our next encounter with the person who angered or upset us, we can say something like, "Can I just go back to something you said yesterday? To be honest I found it a little inappropriate, so do you mind if we discuss this further?" Once we send that emotion back to the person who sparked it in the first place, we can often free ourselves of the pain that it caused.

"I can hardly bear to turn the TV news on; there's so much to be frightened about. Life seems so fragile. It's all I can do to let my kids leave the house. All I want to do is keep them safe from harm."

With so much uncertainty around us in politics and the state of the world, we are overloaded with information about things we are helpless to change but which we take into our own system and add to our emotional load.

For many, this uncertainty can develop into full-blown anxiety, which is what happens when we haven't been listening to our fears. Suddenly, these things take on far too much importance in our minds, and we can feel invaded by all kinds of worries and that we don't have the tools to protect ourselves.

The simplest solution is to remove the source of the information we feel most overloaded by. For example, I make sure that I read the news only once a day, otherwise all that negativity becomes too toxic for me; I also make sure that I read it via a medium that doesn't inflate my fears. Yet all around me I see people's lives interrupted by the latest newsflash or social media update, made available to them day and night, showing them all kinds of bad stuff they didn't really want or need to see. This need to keep oneself informed becomes so addictive that whenever people find themselves with a few spare moments they immediately reach for their devices to get an instant fix.

We all need space to dream, yet we very often don't allow ourselves the privilege. There is nothing wrong with taking time out and letting ourselves feel bored, lonely or even sad. Only when we switch off from the world for a while can we let our minds wander and wonder. We can do this by taking a walk, reading a book, going to an art gallery, watching a movie, or just listening to music or the radio.

I love jazz, so I like to sit and listen and let my mind meander with the notes. I give myself permission to feel good – not guilty – about this time out because I know I'm doing something that's really healthy for my inner balance and that is reconnecting me with my feelings.

SADNESS

"The day Princess Diana died I cried like I haven't cried in years. It was as if a riverbank burst inside me. I couldn't stop thinking about her and her young sons. Afterward, I was exhausted but I also felt strangely relieved."

Sadness is another emotion that is also regarded as negative. But, to my mind, no emotion is negative. Each one is valid and real and should be acknowledged, accepted and understood.

Whenever I come across sadness in a client, together we try to find out where it's coming from before I encourage them to express it. The best way usually is to cry, but some people feel too weak and vulnerable to shed tears and aren't comfortable crying in front of someone else. In which case I suggest instead that they put their feelings down in writing, read back what they've written to help identify their sadness, and then ask themselves a few key questions:

Why am I sad? What happened?

Sadness is very frequently linked with a sense of loneliness, in which case the comfort of food and drink not only acts as an anaesthetic but can also become a companion to rely on – a familiar friend that's always there for us, no matter what. We might feel that everyone around us has abandoned us, let us down or disappointed us in some way, but the sensation of eating a burger and fries, opening a box of chocolates, or drinking a fine wine never disappoints.

What we often don't realize is that it can take a huge amount of time, energy and effort to think about what we're going to eat, when and with whom, and that's before we even start the shopping, the cooking and the enjoying. All of which helps prevent us from thinking about deeper or more painful things. Once we go to the shop or supermarket we can be seized by a kind of emotional frenzy – even eating some of the food we've purchased in the store or on the way home, before getting back to cook and eat the rest.

The focus stays firmly on what we're about to eat, rather than on the sadness that's eating away at our insides far more than any physical hunger. Food becomes yet another distraction, and one that encourages us to overeat, before making us feel bad as we chastise ourselves and tell ourselves – once again – that the diet starts tomorrow.

Have I always been sad, since childhood?

All of us have inner sorrows that no one else knows about, many of which date back to our early years. Remember, I said at the beginning of the book that everyone has a secret. The biggest secret is that we all feel different from everyone else in some way and yet we do our best to fit in and very often hide our true feelings. This is why when people do something dramatic to express or release their pain, those who love them are shocked – because they had no idea how much angst their friend or family member had, and feel guilty that they didn't know.

Was I ever allowed to express my sadness?

There are many reasons why we may be unable to express our sadness. For example, if one of our parents is depressed, then we can't be sad in case it would make the situation worse. We need to ensure that the sadness we're feeling is ours, and not that of someone we care about.

What happens when I do express my sadness?

Strangely, a public sadness like the death of Princess Diana or the events of 9/11 often help people to express their own sorrow in a much more open way. I find that women, and especially mothers, feel far better able to talk about their sadness relating to victims of disasters or public bereavements than they can speak of their own sorrow.

These kinds of public outpourings because of major tragedies or even family funerals can be beneficial for all of us, as they give us permission to let out all those bottled-up feelings and enjoy a rare moment of shared sorrow with friends and strangers.

> **"My father has dementia and gets upset very easily. If I were to start crying or getting upset in front of him, it would tip him over the edge. I've learned to keep a fixed smile on my face and then go somewhere to cry quietly or scream into my hands. Afterward I make myself something to eat."**

So many people who come to see me are afraid to air their sadness in case they accidentally open the floodgates. Their sorrow seems such a huge force within them that they're worried that if they begin to cry they won't be able to stop. Instead they lock up their feelings inside, which will only play tricks on them later.

One middle-aged client whose only sibling died when she was young felt she had to spend her whole life cheering up her parents and being twice the child. Unable to express any strong emotions of her own, she overate to compensate. Even though her parents had also since died, she'd carried on with her unhealthy behaviour.

In a therapy situation like this, I might use what's known as Gestalt Technique, in which the client speaks to an empty chair as if the person he or she needs to hear express their emotions is sitting on it (see opposite). This can create a highly charged scenario, so it ideally needs to be properly supervised.

In this case, I suggested that my client visit the graves of her loved ones and tell them all that she was feeling – even the resentment and anger – and end by telling them how much she loved and missed them. "Speak to them in the way you always wanted to," I suggested. "Let those feelings go."

As with anger, it can also help to write a letter to a person you are missing through death or distance and read it back afterward. You can even write a letter to your sadness. Is it too close a friend? Is it scaring you and taking too much room in your life? You can tell it goodbye for now, and it will leave you alone.

The Gestalt Technique

The Gestalt Technique enables us to connect our thoughts to our feelings and our body in the present moment. This insight – often achieved through role-play – helps us to cut through the confusion and gain a far more realistic vision of who we really are. To repress the pain we experience from trauma or other hurtful incidents, we tend to cut ourselves off from our true selves and fill our heads with a thousand other thoughts. This brain noise can shield us from what we are really feeling. Once we are able to see the situation more clearly and take personal responsibility without the emotional and psychological clamour, we can be more creative in finding solutions and better placed to achieve our goals.

Like everyone, I feel sad sometimes, and when I do I sit somewhere quietly and play a couple of songs that are guaranteed to make me cry. They are both very emotional but one, called *"Dans les yeux de mere"* (In my mother's eyes), reminds me of my late mother and gets me every time.

It is important to do this kind of practice in a safe environment and allow yourself enough privacy and space. Don't do it when you're just about to go out, or on the bus on the way home from work, or when you're surrounded by other people. Sit quietly somewhere on your own, and permit yourself to feel.

If we can't express our sadness even when listening to music or watching a sad movie, then we're in trouble. Unchecked, sadness can lead to depression that often leads to a dependency on alcohol or drugs, and can create long-term mental health problems.

With time and practice, we can learn to cry with serenity because we know in our heart and body that it is doing us some good. Trust me, the days that follow will be lighter.

> **"I can't remember the last time I threw back my head and laughed. The only thing that makes me happy now is macaroni cheese and I mean, a whole dish of it – washed down with red wine. My mum made it whenever I was ill and eating it reminds me of the comfort she gave me."**

We should not quell this flood that seeks to rise in us. Feeling sadness, and accepting it, is far more beneficial than we might think. Whenever I have a client who's in touch with their sadness and starts to cry, I am so pleased for them because I know that they'll soon be able to move forward. The blockage in their emotional system has been cleared.

Often it helps to turn away from the noise and frenzy of life and let this sadness happen. It is an energy that allows us to say farewell, to leave an emotional situation behind before moving on to something else. It is a process through which, after a period of loss or disappointment, we prepare a new version of ourselves.

Sadness doesn't appear as a natural companion in our lives, unfortunately. This is partly because of the societal fear of depression. There are also massive cultural differences, which I see frequently in my clients.

Continental Europeans can express their emotions far more easily than the British, and this loosens their tongues and their tears. I don't judge anybody but it is such a shame, as it is so much easier if you can let these things out. With my British clients, however, I often see grown men sitting with tears in their eyes as long as they can hold on to them, bowing their heads and apologizing. Always apologizing. Americans and Canadians tend to feel constrained by political correctness, which can make it harder to open up about their emotions.

As much as male sadness is frowned upon, it is one of the only emotions allowed to women who, by contrast, are denied the emotion of anger. These emotional diktats don't help anyone and only blur recognition of what's truly happening inside.

The paradox is that, unless we accept someone's sadness with sympathy and understanding, we risk it developing into a depressive state. Experienced in full conscience, with the acceptance that it is a valid emotion, sadness is something that can be seen positively.

"I had no idea how much of my life I was wasting on all these 'negative' emotions until I really started thinking about it. Entire days could pass without one moment of relief. Now I say what I feel when I'm feeling it and the biggest shock of all is that nobody hates me for it after all."

It is only human to feel as if we have failed somehow if we get angry, upset or frightened and haven't been able to control our emotions. This sense of regret only adds to our growing emotional load.

Imagine what we could do with the hours we waste every day on feeling bad or sad, guilty or frustrated, and then all those hours we spend obsessed with feeding ourselves in order to feel better.

Putting our emotions to sleep with food in this way also has a physical effect on our bodies – literally putting us to sleep as our stomachs struggle to digest what we've just consumed. Some people eat or drink late at night specifically to help them fall asleep, but it rarely provides the kind of healthy rest they really need.

Just as when someone is giving up smoking and those around them encourage them to think about all the money they could save, I encourage you to think of all the good things you could be doing instead of eating, thinking about eating, or worrying about your world. Think of it this way:

■ Ask yourself how many minutes in every hour you think about yourself in an emotional or negative way.

■ Add all those minutes when you are thinking about food or your next meal.

■ Incorporate the time wasted worrying about the future in a fearful way.

▓ Finally, add to this score the time spent shopping for and preparing food in a way that is distracting and comforting rather than enjoyable.

▓ Now calculate the final figure, and make a gift of this time to yourself.

If the main benefit of maintaining our unhealthy weight is to put our emotions to sleep by using food, then it's important to have something in place instead. Otherwise we can easily feel overwhelmed by emptiness.

What about learning the piano or the guitar like you always wanted, reading more, learning about your family tree, or doing a long-distance walk? You could do some charity work, take up tennis, join a dance class or a sports team. I started walking everywhere when I first moved to London, and then I started cycling. I use walking therapy with my clients too, strolling around a park together as we talk rather than being confined to a room, a surprisingly uplifting experience for everyone.

The possibilities are endlessly exciting and entirely up to you, so enjoy your new freedom and be creative with the spare time you now have to spend. And if you think you can't afford a new hobby, think about how much you'll save by eating and drinking less: it can be a huge amount!

With the use of simple questions to promote gentle self-awareness, we can unveil exactly what benefits are to be had from not losing the weight we want to. Then we work on changing previously held views and habits, a process that can be truly liberating.

Once you become aware of the mostly unconscious benefits to be had from being overweight and identifying the patterns, I can guide you to eat more intuitively and mindfully.

In order to do this, I will encourage you to open up about your emotions, acknowledge them, and start to manage them more efficiently. These feelings send us important messages and, if we don't take them into consideration, we will frequently use food and alcohol to avoid them or to compensate.

Once again, it will be helpful to ask yourself the following questions about the benefits to you from being overweight, with kindness and without being the Parent (see page 39). Remember this is just a way of getting you to start thinking about your habits and the way you respond.

When you've written down your answers honestly, take time to really think about them, looking at them frequently to build up a picture of yourself that will allow you to see yourself in a mindful, uncritical way.

Do you often consider yourself in negative ways?

If so, what are the words you would use to describe the way you look or behave? Write them down so you can read them back to yourself. Many of my clients tell me that they believe they are greedy or unattractive, selfish or vain. There is so much self-loathing out there.

Take time now to consider how others view you. What kind of image do you think they have of you in general? Do they think you are fat or ugly or self-centred or horrible, the same way that you think of yourself? Most of us believe that our selfishness, greed or vanity is something we are hiding from others, a secret that allows us to keep on pretending to be someone we are not, never showing people who we really are. Do you think people know your secret?

Name five good qualities that would define you.

People find this surprisingly hard to do. Ask yourself questions such as, Am I kind? Do I make my friends laugh? Am I generous with my time, love or money? Do I have a good sense of humour?

Am I a compassionate person? Do people want to be in my company? Can my friends rely on me? Am I good at my job?

Answer these honestly then read the answers back to yourself, out loud. "Yes, I am a good friend. Yes, I am kind. Yes, people find me funny. Yes, I have a good career. I am also very patient." Not all your answers have to be positive, of course, but be realistic.

Reading the answers aloud can often be a revelation. It helps to give us a broader image of who we are and stops us from only seeing the things that we don't achieve, or find hard to do. By seeing the bigger picture and being more realistic about ourselves, we can be the Adult again instead of the judgmental Parent.

Just because you may be carrying more weight than is healthy for you doesn't mean you are a bad person. You may be heavier than you'd like, but it's good to remind yourself that you aren't a racist or a thief, for example. You are a kind, compassionate individual who has been successful at most of the things you have done in your life. Now is the time to stop being so critical of what you see as your failures and focus on your successes. It's good to remind ourselves of our positive aspects once in a while.

Do you think about food all the time and does it take up too much room in your life?

Food is a great comfort and a pleasure, and so it should be. A tasty dinner is something enjoyable to look forward to at the end of the day. But it can also be a lure or a way to fill the emptiness.

Thinking about food, preparing it, eating it and then feeling bad about it is an easy way to procrastinate, or at least to avoid other issues and stop ourselves from moving forward. It reinforces the idea that we are helplessly locked into something that's stronger than us. If we are not careful, we can feel trapped by the whole process.

> **"My obsession has gone far beyond casually browsing through a recipe book or the need to know what to shop for. I must have a clear image in my mind of everything I am going to put into my mouth and know exactly when."**

So many of my clients tell me that the first thing they do when they wake up is think about what they are going to eat at every stage of their day. They have to know what they are going to eat, so that they can count out the hours between meals.

The key is to find some sort of balance between the things you need to do to nourish your body and the rest of your life. It's fine if your thoughts are of straightforward pleasure in looking forward to the opening of a new restaurant or a night out with friends. You might think, "Oh, it's curry night tonight. I think I'll have that delicious tandoori prawn dish I had last time," or, "I'll grab a quick bite on the way home and then I won't have to cook."

The problem is that it is unusual for people to think freely about these things and then forget about them. Thoughts about food invade every aspect of their day until they feel as if the thoughts are on a loop in their brains. They start to obsess about the quantities, the calories, and how much they are going to eat and drink. It's all mapped out in advance as they set themselves up for a fall.

Using my examples from above, they might think, "Oh, it's curry night tonight. I think I'll have that delicious tandoori prawn dish I had last time – and a few poppadoms, and maybe some onion bhajis and a couple of cold beers to wash it down." Or, "I'll grab a quick bite in the pub on the way home and then I won't have to cook. If my mates are there, I suppose I'll stay for a pint or two, eat some savoury snacks before my burger, and then maybe on the way home I'll pick up some ice cream."

They haven't given enough consideration to how hungry they might be, or whether a curry or a burger is the healthiest thing for them to eat. Instead, they are planning for indulgence and looking forward to it, even though they know that the following day they'll probably be wracked with guilt about how much they ate or drank.

"Whenever I'm eating something I shouldn't, it's like I flick a switch in my head that turns off the me that knows it's wrong. That switch only flicks back on again the next morning, when I slide out of bed with a groan like a naughty child."

All these obsessional thoughts can start to feel like a mission we have to accomplish. Our procrastination means we don't really succeed in our most important project, such as fixing a relationship (or ending one), making a career change, or spending more quality time with those we love. Our universe becomes defined by when and how much we can eat, and then by how overweight we are.

When we ask ourselves what we can replace these food projects with that would be more enjoyable or beneficial, we are often lost for suggestions. Many of us have been addicted to food for such a long time that we don't even know what we would do if we could make more time for ourselves. We cannot imagine having all that free mental headspace when we can just enjoy food and not think about it a hundred times a day.

Give yourself the permission to try to free yourself from the food loop. Imagine a world where what you are going to eat and every detail of your interaction with it doesn't take that much room anymore. Just imagine, within a few months you can live in that world; a place where you are simply happy to be going to a restaurant and won't think about the menu until it's in your hand.

Can you see yourself as that person, with that much mental free time? It's a scary question for many, but – together – we can do it.

TO RECAP

- Think of the benefits that you gain from being overweight.

- Are you using food to quash unwanted emotions and put yourself to sleep?

- Remember, we are all of us carrying an emotional load.

- Anger, fear and sadness can overwhelm us if we let them, so pay attention to these valid emotions and express them in a healthy way.

- Using food to put these emotions to sleep leads only to bigger problems later on.

- Clear the brain noise and connect to your thoughts in the present moment.

- Replace your negative feelings with positive ones and think of all the things you could be enjoying instead of wasting time with dark, unhappy thoughts.

CASE STUDY

When I was overweight, I came to realize that there were aspects of being heavy that suited me. I wasn't poor before I met my wife, but being married to her elevated me to a whole new status. She was a textile designer and her family was wealthy. Instead of the simple holidays on a Greek island that I was accustomed to, she would rent a luxurious suite on an island in the Caribbean. Instead of my small apartment on the outskirts of Brussels, we lived in a beautiful house right in the centre.

We no longer went to the same kind of restaurants and, although I loved my life and everyone considered me very lucky, having so much money wasn't really me. I wanted to fit in, so I started reinventing myself. No one asked me to do that, but to survive emotionally I had to create a new persona – which wasn't the real me either.

I have always been a people pleaser, so by inviting friends over to eat and cooking for them I felt that I was taking care of them somehow. I would often slave all day over a meal and then busy myself making sure that everyone was getting along with each other and having a good time. It took so much energy and I secretly felt I had to work so hard to please them all.

About five years into my marriage I started gaining weight for the first time in my life and – over a long period – I gained 30 kilos (5 stone). I was aware of how unhealthy it was and I wanted it to stop, but I didn't do anything serious about it because psychologically I needed to put the weight on. My wife and friends commented about my weight occasionally but never in a nasty way, and I often made a joke of it too. I had a best mate who was as heavy as me and our friends loved having the two of us over for dinner, knowing that we would eat heartily and with relish.

Before too long I was busy running two restaurants in Brussels, but there were problems. Because I always tried to be kind and helpful to everyone, I now appreciate that I exacerbated these problems with my compassion and empathy rather than solving them using assertiveness. The situation made me feel only more trapped and unhappy, and I was too busy helping everyone else to take care of myself. Frustrated and angry, scared about the future and feeling stuck in life, I ate even more to mask my loneliness and dull the pain.

I made a few feeble attempts to lose weight and I even went to a gym, but I hated seeing myself in a mirror and didn't like being surrounded by so many fit, slim people. Plus, I was too tired and physical exercise hurt too much, so I gave up.

My wife and I grew apart, becoming more like friends than lovers. We went to see an excellent therapist who helped me understand myself better for the first time. He made me realize I was spending too much of my energy being good to everyone. I used my weight to avoid being intimate, and our marriage eventually failed the year my mother died, a few years after my father. It had lasted 16 years and produced two wonderful children, so I have no regrets, and now my wife and I are very good friends.

3

WHY DO YOU REPEATEDLY SABOTAGE YOURSELF?

"I'm my own worst enemy. It's as if I have a devil on my shoulder telling me I've never succeeded in the past and I'll never do it this time either, so why am I even trying?"

Just as I did, many of us struggle with our body image for years. This struggle can become a defining part of us – a way to describe ourselves to others. Whatever great qualities we may have can be dwarfed by these inner feelings of insecurity.

Once we've understood that there may be subconscious reasons for remaining overweight, then we can start to work on cancelling out the many ways in which we repeatedly sabotage our attempts to change the way we look. This is something we do because we're afraid that losing weight will expose us in some way – physically or emotionally – and take us to a new and scary place where we may not feel so invisible. If we are overeating to avoid anger or loneliness, guilt or confrontation, fear or sadness, then what happens to those emotions when we stop overeating? How on earth will we be able to face them?

By examining the emotional and psychological issues underlying this phenomenon, we can explain the extent to which mostly unconscious issues drive our eating habits and why we continually undermine ourselves. By being mindful about our hunger, and excavating the causes of the problem, we can allow ourselves to make changes for good. We will see how best to harness our emotions so that they no longer take control of our eating.

I hear so many excuses from clients who repeatedly sabotage their plans to lose weight that I could probably write a book just about them. Apart from the kinds of reasons we have already dealt with about comfort eating or quashing unwanted emotions, they come up with all sorts of inventive ideas: "If I lose weight I'll spend the rest of my life worrying about putting it back on," or, "It's going to take so long, and I won't be able to enjoy life anymore," or, "I'm not a good person. I need to punish myself."

Even those who commit to their decision to lead a healthier way of life and try to lose weight can start to create reasons why they've had a lapse or can't continue. "It's hopeless. I weighed myself today and I've already gained two of the five pounds I lost!"

In the process of losing weight, weighing ourselves makes complete sense. I believe it's something we should do once a week to make sure that we're on the right path. It should always be done in the morning, using the same scales and without any clothes on.

This may seem logical, but many of my clients seem to forget this, or use it as a way to find an excuse to give up. Some of us are almost allergic to scales and will choose instead to estimate our weight loss by how comfortable we feel in our clothes, but this can play tricks on us if our clothes have shrunk slightly through washing or loosened through wear. An alternative is to measure different parts of our body such as our chest, hips and thighs, but I still think that the scales are the best way to find out if we're making progress in the right direction.

If we become unhealthily fixated on our weight, stepping on the scales several times a day – which many of my clients do – can only lead to disappointment and reinforce a negative feeling that we won't succeed. It's not unusual for some people to use their scales, not as an indicator, but to confirm how "bad" they have been. In their mind's eye, the scales can also become the Parent (see page 39), chastising them for not losing enough or putting weight back on. They can punish themselves by standing before the scales the morning after they've eaten too much, knowing that the sight of the accusatory reading will be their penance.

This kind of behaviour only helps feed the negative image we might already have of ourselves. We are too greedy. We're a failure. This, in turn, makes us feel angry and sad. It is yet another method of sabotage that can trap us into giving up. We have to give ourselves permission to carry on, regardless, and remind ourselves that we may have lost one battle, but not the war.

The truth is that if we eat a heavy meal, or snack on something fattening, and gain one or two pounds as a consequence, it isn't the end of the world. We can lose it again quite quickly with a bit of thought. We just have to use the tools we have already learned about choosing what we eat and when, slowing down, and savouring our food up until the point when we have had enough.

Yet the excuses keep coming. At the end of every session, I ask my clients, "What is in the way of you losing another three or four pounds before we meet again?" I often see their faces cloud over or their foreheads wrinkle into a frown as they start to lay themselves traps in order to fail.

"Oh, this is going to be a very difficult week for me. I have business lunches or dinners every day, and I can't get out of any of them. How can I say no to wine or to dessert when my client is asking if we can have a second bottle or wants to order a soufflé?"

"That's no problem," I reply with a smile. "Eating out is an excellent way to lose weight. You don't have to cook or handle the food. You have so many things to choose from on a menu. There are always healthy options, and you can ask for a smaller portion or just leave what you don't want on your plate. As for drinking, you can enjoy a couple of glasses if you feel like it and then stop."

Once again, a little forward planning here is often all it takes to prepare for these occasions. If you are hungry then eat something light and healthy before your meal. This will allow you to eat more slowly and consume less once you are at the restaurant.

Few see it as being that simple, though. For many, going out to eat in a restaurant is a treat for a special or rare occasion and they feel entitled to indulge. They can even feel aggrieved if they think they can't choose the food they want. "But the desserts there are so delicious and I really don't know if I can say no."

"Okay," I reply, "but who said you should avoid dessert? Avoid having a starter instead and select something healthy as a main. Try to make sure that your previous meal and the one afterward are also healthier. None of us puts on weight with just one meal."

Then there are all the other pitfalls. Waiting staff are trained to encourage us to have a starter and a dessert as well as a main. We can't blame them for that; they're just doing their job. But we shouldn't order more food than we need just to please them, because it will be us who pays for the consequences. The same goes for drinks. Don't feel bad if you're only ordering one glass of wine or a jug of tap water. Alcohol is a big money-spinner for the hospitality business but it can be a significant hurdle on our path to weight loss. Don't hesitate to tell your waiter you don't want him to keep filling your wine glass.

Another issue I often encounter with clients eating out is that when they are paying for a meal they consider it a waste of money to leave any food on their plate. Yet the food we don't eat represents very little of what we spend. We are paying far more for the pleasure of eating out in a pleasant environment with full service and no need to prepare it or wash up afterward. Overeating in that scenario is even more wasteful than any financial loss, because, even though our body is telling us it has had enough, we still think it's better to finish the food rather than have it thrown away. We are effectively using our body as a bin, which is a waste of the food, with untold long-term costs to our health. Plus it takes away all the pleasure if you are going to feel guilty of overeating afterward.

Many of my clients fall into the trap of ordering more food or drink merely to extend the pleasure of an enjoyable time in a restaurant with family or friends. I hear it all around me whenever I eat out: "Let's order another bottle of wine," or, "Who's going to join me in dessert?" or, "Come on, have something. It's a special occasion. I know you're trying to watch your weight but you can be good tomorrow."

This is fine if we fully appreciate what we're doing and make sure we leave something on our plate. But whenever we do leave food, we should be prepared for the additional pressure restaurant staff can put us under. They often appear disappointed and ask if something was wrong with the meal. In this situation, we start apologizing and feel as though we have to justify our action, when we only have to justify our behaviour to ourselves.

Habits like these can be difficult to change, but once we've broken them once or twice we will begin to wonder why we thought it would be so difficult. I know it can sound hard or even boring not to allow ourselves to overindulge so frequently with food and drink, but that's simply because we're not used to behaving this way.

Meals out are never the reason we might eat or drink too much. It is much more about how we feel in that situation. Who are we with? Are we bored, or maybe wishing we were somewhere else? Do we feel we are being judged on what we say or do? How do we cope with being poured some more wine or being asked to share a dessert? Is there peer group pressure to join in when we don't want to? Remember:

It's not about the dinner.

It's never about the food.

It's about our emotional insecurities.

Eating in can be just as easy to blame as eating out. For example, I hear so many mothers tell me, "The kids were with their father this week and I missed them, so I ate and drank too much to compensate." Or the very next parent I see might say, "I had to take care of the children this half-term and I ended up eating twice because I cooked for them first, picking at the food, and then I sat down to eat with my partner when he came home from work."

I hear people tell me that their food scales were broken, so they roughly estimated how much something weighed only to discover later that they'd eaten twice what they'd meant to. Or, "The recipe I was using said to add 150 grams of cheese but I misread it as 250. It tasted really good, though!"

Eating up leftovers seems to present a huge temptation too, especially if there is some cold pizza left in the box, or extra food from dinner out the night before, wrapped up and taken home. If a child or other family member leaves half a burger, some fish fingers or fries on their plate, there is a high chance that a parent will finish it off for them – rather than throw it away – without considering the fact that they aren't really hungry or have just eaten themselves. Not to mention snacks and cookies left lying around. How quick and easy it is to grab a handful and eat it so quickly that you don't even have the chance to think about how many extra calories it might add up to. The same goes for that quarter bottle of wine left over after a party.

Then there are all the Sunday lunches and other family meals, the birthday and wedding celebrations. Not to mention the corporate events and leaving parties – and Christmas, the biggest temptation of all. My goodness, the "season of goodwill" seems to be such a big hurdle to overcome for anyone who wants to lose weight. There is goodwill, it seems, for everyone but ourselves.

"Well, it was Christmas and we had one party after another, plus the blowout dinner with turkey and all the trimmings. I knew there was no way I would lose weight. I'm just grateful I only gained 5 pounds."

We can always find excuses to overeat or overdrink in any situation, but they are just that – excuses, none of which is valid. I don't judge anyone for that. I just want you to understand what is going on and why these triggers can set you on the wrong path. Only then can you learn to identify the triggers and stop sabotaging yourself. Feeling guilty about it is counterproductive.

It is time to acknowledge responsibility.

One of the things I find so interesting is that we very often judge ourselves so very harshly, and in a far less forgiving way than we do others, such as our friends or relatives. Why do we have so much more empathy and compassion for those around us than we do for ourselves? Imagine that you have a dear friend who is kind and compassionate, caring and selfless, but who happens to be a bit overweight. Would it make any difference to your relationship with him or her? Would you even notice or care? Probably not.

And yet you will happily stand in front of a mirror and make disgusted faces because you don't like your own body shape or size, and never even take into account what a fine person you are. When you see your own reflection, you completely overlook the fact that you are a great friend, a good mum or dad and a terrific colleague, and often put others before yourself. Your weight, shape or size has nothing to do with any of that, but if you want to make changes then – guess what? – you are the one person who is best placed to do so. I would even argue that you have an ethical and moral obligation to look after yourself before you look after others. It's a bit like fitting your own oxygen mask on a plane before helping anyone else – only when you can breathe will you be useful to others.

If we can only build a better image of ourselves in our minds, one that reflects who we really are, then we can start to be kinder to that person, more respectful, and maybe even love them a little.

Sabotage is something we have all become expert at, so this kind of self-compassion and self-acceptance is our best ally in losing the extra weight for once and for all. Now might be the time to ask yourself some questions about your own reasons for repeatedly undermining yourself.

As before, take time to carefully consider your answer and then write down your answers and read them aloud to yourself. Reflect on what you have come up with, and return to the answers regularly as a way of reminding yourself how you felt when you wrote them, and compare it to how you feel then.

Can you allow yourself to believe that things might change for good?

If the honest answer is no, then ask yourself why not. Is it because you have unkindly labelled yourself as not having enough willpower or courage, or being too greedy? Think back and try to remember if there was someone in your life, such as a parent or parent-figure, who said you were like that.

Is it possible that your belief about your guaranteed failure originated from that person? If that is the case, then let go of the Child in you, take responsibility, and become the Adult. Accept that this sense of failure comes from someone else in the past and not from you. Understand that their reasons for labelling you in that way might well have come from their own insecurities and emotional deficiencies. They may even have been trying to forewarn you about their own inadequacies and disappointments.

I don't believe in laziness or greed. I think it's much more about being blocked emotionally and not giving ourselves the right to do what we know is best for us.

Can you imagine yourself in five years' time?

What do you see? To make it more realistic, estimate how old you will be and if you'll still be in the same job, or if your kids will have left school. To begin with, try to imagine that you have lost all the weight you want and have made long-lasting changes to your life. You look great and have so much more confidence. You feel loved, cherished and understood, and generally feel so much better about yourself.

Now, imagine the other scenario – that five years have passed and there has been no change. Perhaps you have gained even more weight, going up three sizes. You are older now, with far more pressing health issues that will have a direct correlation to your weight. You are unhappier than ever: still trapped in a body you feel ashamed of; still locked into the job, relationship or situation that made you sad, frightened, angry or lonely in the first place.

Which is more scary? The option where you have to focus on your goals for a relatively short period of time to achieve the future you both want and deserve? Or a situation where you are spiralling into further weight gain with bigger health problems in an emotional space where you are unhappier than you are now? Ask yourself which is the riskier option. Deciding to make the changes I am encouraging you to make now, or the scenario of what will undoubtedly happen if you do nothing at all?

Know that I respect your fears. I, of all people, understand that it isn't easy to make these changes. But if you really want to prevent the second option from coming true, then this is what we have to do – together.

"I can't ever imagine myself being happy with my weight. It's like a mental block. I keep all my old clothes in my wardrobe 'just in case' I ever slim down enough to get into them again, but every time I see them I just feel depressed because it seems like an impossible task."

What is it that you are really scared of?

Whenever we sabotage our attempts to lose weight we also undermine our hopes of moving forward with our lives. The extra kilos or pounds we carry can become like an anchor, weighing us down and preventing us from going in the right direction.

We become fearful of the unknown, especially of what our weight loss might mean for us and those around us.

Ask yourself:

- Will it mean that I have to deprive myself for a long period of time and never be able to fully enjoy a social situation again?

- Will being slimmer change the way I interact with others, or the way others respond to me?

- Is this the right time to embark on such a major change in my way of life, or should I wait until I am better prepared?

If you take a moment to consider all these fears, you'll find that losing weight mindfully isn't scary or dangerous at all. If you want to know what will really happen when you reach your healthy weight, the answer is not much, apart from the fact that you'll feel healthier, better looking and much more confident. You will have more energy and enjoy feeling generally better about yourself. This is great news and nothing to be scared of at all.

Being slimmer doesn't mean that you will become a different person or that your life will change dramatically. Many of my clients have a distorted image of what will happen, based on the people they know or see in the media who are slim. They often think of such people as arrogant, selfish or vain, but there's no basis for this other than envy or a mistaken belief.

Instead of discovering a *new* you, you'll be connecting with the *real* you.

Of course, there may be some around you who feel confronted or threatened by the change in you, either because they're also struggling with food issues or because – for whatever reason – they feel reassured by seeing you overweight, but that's their issue. It shouldn't be yours.

Then there are those who fear that being slim again will only remind them of their youth – a time when they felt free sexually. They worry that their weight loss might encourage them back into situations that could be inappropriate or risky for their existing relationship. Believe me, none of my clients has become a sex addict after losing weight, but almost all of them have improved their sex lives with their partners by gaining more confidence.

For those without a partner for whatever reason, there is often the fear that their weight loss will put them "back on the market" and force them into the terrors of a new relationship. The idea of this can be very frightening if you have experienced emotional pain in the past. Losing weight doesn't mean that you will automatically meet someone new straightaway, however. You can take your time, see how you feel, engage with others, look back at those painful past relationships with the eyes of the Adult in you. Life doesn't have to be about repeating your mistakes over and over again. If you choose to be in a relationship, then remember that you deserve to be in a benevolent one without having to pay an emotional price.

Things are more difficult for those who have been abused. The extra weight they carry can become an emotional and physical shield, and to lose that can be very frightening. If it proves too much of a hurdle, then I recommend professional help in order to feel fully supported and safe while losing weight. People tend to stick to what is familiar, even if it means staying in an uncomfortable comfort zone.

> **"My partner does everything for me around the house these days because I'm so heavy and can't easily get around anymore. He's wonderful and I can't imagine how I would cope without him."**

What is your overweight "persona"? Is it this you are afraid to lose?

When I was carrying all that extra weight, I didn't appreciate that it had become so much a part of me that I had built a whole persona around it. I pretended to be always happy, always smiling, always energetic. Remember, I was a pleaser and – as such – my only option seemed to be to show a positive image of myself.

I even became a stand-up comedian, doing "improv" at a national and international level, using my weight as a prop to play the fat king or the jolly landlord. I didn't want anyone to think that I was suffering in any way from being overweight, or know how much pain I was in. I can still remember how draining it was to keep up that fake persona.

Others can use their extra weight similarly to create a "victim persona" in which their lives revolve around their size in a negative way. They complain all the time about their condition and the attendant health issues. In this kind of scenario, they very often bond with those who come to regard themselves as their "saviours" – people who think that worrying for others, taking care of them, and even feeding them is somehow loving them.

That isn't loving, though.

These "saviours" often have their own issues, in which the only way they feel they can become close to others is to be needed. They may well also be overweight. That's not love but a kind of codependence. Those who can live only through a dependent relationship will always seek someone to worry about and take care of. What this means for the person who is obese is that losing a large amount of weight for health and emotional reasons could seriously jeopardize their relationship with their saviour. In that situation, the question you have to ask yourself is, "Do I want to carry that weight for the rest of my life just to protect my partner and not risk losing them, or do I want to have a more balanced, healthier relationship?"

In younger people this type of unhealthy codependence can develop in the relationship with one or both parents. Weight can become the main subject of discussion between them, so that by continually overeating and keeping the status quo, the child maintains the equilibrium of the relationship. It is not uncommon to see obese parents living with obese children, with whom they share a common physical and emotional bond. The danger is that the child will be too afraid to break away and live a different kind of life.

Being a dependant or codependant like this is often not a conscious choice, but it can still create fear and lead to unintentional sabotage. No one is going to consciously think, "I'd better keep Mum and Dad busy with my weight issues or they might feel useless, fall into depression, or even get divorced," but I can see how and why some people come to think that. What I try to tell them is that the parents of my younger clients have only ever expressed delight and relief when their children were able to lose weight and gain a new level of independence.

Most of these kinds of scenario go back to our childhood, when we either relished our dependence on the adults in our lives – and were therefore reluctant to give it up – or when we developed some kind of idea that it was our "mission" to save our parents once we grew up. In every case, the healthiest first step is to recognize that we are not children anymore. We are adults – as are those around us – and each of us is responsible for our own life.

It may be hard to see this at first, but the reality is that the consequences of us losing weight are far less significant for others than we might think. The people around us genuinely do not think as much about our size and shape as we do. How could anyone?

Weight loss does not lead to a revolution but to an evolution. It allows us to lead a better life and make peace with ourselves, and to accept that we are not responsible for the happiness of others, and that it is no longer our role to protect others from dealing with their own issues.

Are you overeating to punish yourself for something?

We live in a world that can be very unforgiving, one in which we are expected to fit into all kinds of norms and behave in certain ways. Society and our education tell us how we should behave and what we should think and believe. But the human mind is very complex and doesn't always find its place that easily.

Whenever we are feeling or behaving in a way that doesn't conform, we can become afraid of our thoughts and fantasies and start to believe that we're not as good as we should be. Many have the feeling that they are hiding their true self as a secret inside and feel ashamed. Some people even see themselves as wicked or bad.

"Other people think I'm a good person, but if they knew who I really am and what I really think, they wouldn't believe it. I'm a terrible person. I sometimes wish I'd never had children. I envy my friends when good things happen to them. I eat and drink my way through the day and think horrible thoughts."

Some believe that they weren't good children and that they are the real reason for their parents' depression or divorce. Others hate themselves for not being able to satisfy their partners sexually and convince themselves that it is only a matter of time before they'll be left on their own. A few blame themselves for some tragedy or incident that shocked the family and altered its dynamic. Many carry the secret of a one-night stand after they had drunk too much, terrified that the truth will come out. The examples are countless, but all of them reflect the immense amount of guilt some carry on their shoulders.

In this scenario it is common to sabotage any attempts to lose weight by overeating and drinking too much as a kind of punishment. If people feel "ugly" inside, they feel as if they have to pay for that and be "ugly" outside too. They see themselves as misfits. They may not sabotage themselves consciously, of course, but unless they realize this pattern then the multiple failures they face in their attempts to lose weight will only reinforce this negative image of themselves.

It is important to understand that, to a certain extent, we are all misfits trying to find our place in this world. Everyone around us feels the same way. It is unfair to punish ourselves just because we're struggling to be at peace with who we are, or with the inner thoughts or fantasies we might have. Losing weight won't work if it means going into battle with ourselves. We have to accept that we aren't perfect – nobody is – and be comfortable with who we are.

Self-compassion and acceptance are our best allies on that path. If we have really done something wrong or hurt someone, then it is probably best to apologize or see if we can fix things. Envy of friends who are doing better than us is very common – especially if they have more money, a smarter house or a better-looking partner. And the burden of trying to be a perfect parent, perfect partner or perfect child is too much for anyone to bear.

If we can only think more kindly about ourselves and others, despite our many flaws, then we can truly begin to appreciate that everyone else is struggling too. As an exercise to help this, try the following:

- Write down the name of a person in your life that you like and admire but also envy. Now list the reasons why you envy them, followed by the reasons why you like them. Are they kind to you and others? Do they make you laugh? Are they generous with themselves? Would they help you out in a crisis? Focus on their positive qualities and remind yourself why they are in your life.

- Next, write down the name of someone you have hurt or have been unkind to in the past. Think back to the reasons you did that and how much time you have wasted dwelling on what you did. Was it justified? Did you do it in the heat of the moment? Do you still regret the way you behaved? Now compose an apology to them, trying to explain why you behaved in that way. If you feel able, send them the apology, or tell them face to face, even if the events you are addressing happened a long time ago.

- If you feel that you have been trying too hard to be a perfect parent, the perfect husband or wife, or the perfect child or friend, then write down how that makes you really feel inside.

Inadequate? A fraud? As if you are living a lie? Write down your own doubts and weaknesses with regard to that relationship and really think about them now. Are you too controlling? Is that because this relationship is the only thing you really feel in control of? Have you been hiding your doubts and fears? Write them down now and think of ways in which you might start to show the softer side of yourself – the real you – with all your flaws. Imagine how liberating it would feel not to search for perfection all the time but to be able to say, "I'm sorry, I didn't have a great day today and I would love it if you would help me with something."

Being authentically you will give you safe ground on which to move forward with your life and let you stop feeling like a fraud. Remember, we are all of us misfits, trying to do the best we can. What you need to do now is forgive yourself and move on to become the person you truly want to be.

Think how many ways you have sabotaged yourself recently when it came to overeating. What was your best excuse to yourself or others? And your worst? Doing this will help you to see that each day brings new opportunities to undermine yourself.

In the next chapter we will discuss the people who surround you and how they impact on your self-perception and confidence, but take a moment here to consider whether your frequent self-sabotage might partly be to maintain the status quo with those you live with.

Use this new insight to accept that you and you alone are responsible for everything about you: your body, your mind, everything that comes out of your mouth and everything that goes into it. Look at yourself anew with compassion, kindness and courage. Acknowledge that there are aspects of yourself that you may like less than others, but choose now to face those aspects with hope and gentleness and to change them for the better at your own pace.

Remind yourself of your finest qualities and the strength and determination that have enabled you to survive all that life has thrown at you so far. There is no one else in the world who has had your life experiences or who thinks just like you. All that you do is authentically yours. You alone can choose to change the way you behave. You have already started. Remember, it is you who chose to read this book. So, let's keep going.

TO RECAP

● Change is scary, so we often sabotage our weight loss to avoid facing the consequences of being more exposed.

● Don't become unhealthily fixated on how much weight you are losing or gaining.

● Give yourself permission to fail occasionally, but learn from these failures and then carry on with your plan.

● Stop making excuses for yourself and take responsibility for what goes into your mouth.

● Allow yourself to believe that things will change for the better and imagine yourself in five years' time.

● Connect with the real you and behave authentically, not as your "persona".

● Focus on your positive qualities and develop them.

CASE STUDY

Simone is an attractive woman who comes from a wealthy, middle-class family that was rather rigid and controlling. As a teenager she rebelled, leaving home to embrace the punk movement and embark on a promiscuous way of life in which she had many lovers. She repeatedly described her old self as "a slut" or "a bitch".

When she accidentally fell pregnant with her first child, she married young, but she and her new husband both continued to have affairs with others throughout their tempestuous marriage. After they divorced, she was left alone to raise her child and continued to have many boyfriends until she met her second husband, with whom she fell in love and had another child.

Eager to make her second marriage work, Simone didn't tell her husband about her former life as she felt "ashamed" and it was her secret. Being with him, though, helped her "go back to factory settings", as she put it. She became a dutiful and loving wife and mother but quickly started to gain weight, sabotaging every attempt she made to control her overeating. Being overweight became a kind of security blanket for her, matching what she regarded as the "mumsy" woman she had now become.

Referring to her past as "the dark days", she had a real and genuine fear that there was a wicked side to her personality that might return her to her former promiscuousness if she were to become slim and - as she saw it - more attractive again. Subconsciously, she cushioned herself against that psychologically and physically by gaining a large amount of weight.

During her wilder days she had felt judged by her parents all the time, and that only made her rebel more. Now that she was a wife and a parent with a family of her own, she was judging herself just as harshly, hating herself for events long past.

With gentle coaxing, I was able to help her understand that, while it is okay to regret certain aspects of our earlier lives, it isn't healthy or fair to punish ourselves for them forever. For some reason, she had been looking for love as a younger woman and was in a lot of pain. We are all of us looking for love. She may have gone about it in a different way from most but now – with her Adult ego state – she could forgive the Child and stop being the Parent, constantly judging herself.

"You are not that person anymore," I told her. "You have changed and only you can decide how you behave now." I helped her let go of the past, free herself from the guilt and shame, and embrace a new life in which she could be anything she wanted to be. With time, Simone gradually lost all the weight she wanted to lose, and it was such a revelation to her that she could be all that she wanted to be as a woman, a wife and a mother, and not be overweight.

4

WHY CARE SO MUCH ABOUT WHAT OTHERS THINK?

"When I lost all the weight my partner said the best thing of all wasn't how much better I looked physically but how much healthier I was emotionally. I had no idea how depressing and exhausting it had been for him to hear me talking about food and how fat I was all the time."

We all live within networks. By networks I mean the groups of people who form the different parts of our lives. There is our close family, our extended family, our friends, our work environment, and our relationships with our lovers or partners, all of whom are pivotal to our sense of self-worth. All of these networks together form another, larger network.

In this chapter, we will be focusing on something called Systemic Therapy, where we will examine the social systems in which we all live and how our actions, including our decision to lose weight, might impact on these and the relationships within them (see opposite). These days, this often includes the social networks that so many of us are connected to and in which we receive almost immediate feedback from other people by a "like" or a thumbs-up, and what effect these – or the absence of them – can have on us psychologically.

These networks can play tricks on us in our attempts to lose weight. Only when we understand the difference between how we think others regard us and how we're actually seen can we address these issues, and turn them into networks that support and reinforce rather than challenge our healthy eating.

This aspect of the therapy also touches on the Transactional Analysis I have already spoken about – the way in which we communicate with others and even ourselves on three different levels of ego state – Parent, Adult or Child (see page 39). For example, if I eat too much then the Adult in me will tell me I ate too much, the Parent will judge and admonish me, and the rebellious Child will say, "I don't care, I'm going to have dessert."

The ideal is to think mostly as an Adult if possible, although we need our inner Child to be creative, to make jokes and to make love. My goal is for you to become responsible for your own actions, desires and responses within the boundaries of these different ego states in a way that is respectful and gentle.

If I were to address you as a Parent then you might respond as a Child, which is why I always interact with my clients as an Adult speaking to an Adult.

Systemic Therapy

Systemic Therapy helps us to think of ourselves not solely as individuals but also as people within relationships who have to interact on a daily basis with those around us – in our families and at work, with our friends and our wider social circle. It advocates that individuals should not be viewed in isolation but rather within various systems, such as the family, as well as within work systems and those relating to a social life. By understanding the ripple effect that anything we do or change can have on the group or "system" as a whole, we are able to see that the responses and reactions of others within that group can have an impact on our own decision-making and behaviour.

All of us have strong beliefs (some of them subconscious) about how others perceive us. We might decide that people think of us as lazy or greedy whenever we are carrying too much weight. We may imagine that they consider us lacking in ambition, energy or self-respect. Believe it or not, even though we may dislike what others think of us, the truth is that we might actually be getting some kind of benefit from this perception.

If we think people consider us lazy, then that gives us permission to conform to the stereotype and be a little lazier than we might otherwise be. "I might as well be hung for a sheep as a lamb" is the age-old saying, so what's the point in volunteering to do a bit of extra work, staying later or taking on someone else's load, if people assume we never would?

The same goes for the perception of being the greedy one in a network. If we are convinced that everyone already thinks we are "greedy pigs" with no willpower or self-respect, then we might as well help ourselves to that second slice of cake and enjoy it. What do we have to lose? For some people, overeating has become part of their persona and is how they are defined.

Similarly, if a host or hostess has become known for always "putting on a good spread" at their home, heaping the dinner table with food and encouraging everyone to eat more, then to change their ways would mean stopping all that and might be believed to affect their whole way of socializing.

Then there is the member of the obese family who feels trapped by intergenerational patterns. Perhaps you want to lose weight, but you have tried every diet without success and you feel repeatedly sabotaged by your partner or loved ones. It isn't that your family don't love you, but they are too afraid to make the change with you and would rather things stayed the same because it feels "safe" and "comfortable".

What all this means is that, when we finally take control of our eating habits and start to lose weight, we can face a new and hitherto unexpected problem – that of the image we project of ourselves to others within our systems and networks. It can feel very scary to suddenly become the slim, fit one in a family or social situation, the motivated energetic colleague at work, or the host who offers healthier options at the barbecue.

What would the consequences of that be? How might our loved ones, friends and colleagues react?

> **"I have three sisters-in-law who are all much younger than me and dress in tight sexy outfits while I lived in baggy black clothes for years. Once I started to lose weight, I felt like dressing differently and I could immediately tell that they felt challenged and unsettled by my new look."**

What often happens in these situations within our networks is that we sabotage ourselves in some way by having preconceptions about how others will react to the new version of ourselves.

By asking yourself a few important questions and really considering your answers, you can override this natural tendency and find a way through the labyrinth of anxiety that may well be the product of your own insecurity. The following exercise will help you to do this:

- Find somewhere comfortable to sit and close your eyes. Imagine yourself being slim and see yourself within your various networks, walking around each situation in your mind. See yourself at home with your family or partner; at work with colleagues; and in a social situation with friends.

- Analyse what could happen in these situations, and voice your concerns out loud – even if your fears and perceptions may seem silly or sound awkward when addressing them.

- To make it more realistic, imagine yourself slim in those same networks in three months' time, then in six months, and finally in a year.

- Will you dress differently? Is your hairstyle or your general appearance going to be changed from the one you have now?

- Will you start to move your body in another way? Will you feel sexier, more alive and energetic?

- Will you have more confidence? Will you look at others like you do now?

- When you see that new you in the future and then think of yourself now, do you feel that you may have built a persona that revolves around your extra weight? If so, how do you feel about that?

- Once you have an image of yourself in the future, consider what impact this might have in the systems around you – good and bad. Will your partner be jealous, or feel like being more intimate? Will your children see you as a role model, or as competition? Will people at work treat you with more or less respect? How will strangers judge you?

This exercise isn't easy, as you may find it difficult to remain focused long enough. I would recommend you take notes and read them later on. You don't have to address all the systems at the same time but make sure you do the exercise with all of them.

Many of us might feel tempted to project negative images of ourselves in these future situations, already judging ourselves (as the Parent), and imagining that people are talking about us behind our backs (the Child). When we do this we are just setting ourselves up for a fall, so we need to look at the bigger picture, through the eyes of the Adult.

At times when we are overweight we may have the feeling that we're somehow hiding behind our body image – or at least that we're hiding a part of ourselves. If we fear that by losing weight we will unveil the real person that nobody truly knows, then this idea can be quite scary. The solution lies in not judging ourselves so unfairly and placing less pressure on our shoulders. We all have our very own fantasies and fears – it is what makes us human.

For example, being overweight can be the perfect excuse not to be proactive in finding a partner. If we have a history of difficult or abusive relationships, feeling unhappy with our own bodies is a simple way to place ourselves off circuit. It's another way of subconsciously sabotaging our dreams of being in a relationship.

If this is the case for you, then make a deal with yourself. Tell yourself, I am going to be slim, but I still won't be ready to start dating again. I'll wait until I have solved my relationship issues, but in the meantime I will not sacrifice my health and wellbeing. Only then will I be open to the idea of dating again with much more self-confidence.

"What if my friends and family don't like the real me? Or think that person isn't as good as they think I am now? The truth is that the real me is frightened and angry and jealous and has lots of dark thoughts, all hidden behind a fake smile."

Think for a moment how much time you waste worrying about what other people think of you – at work with your colleagues and clients, and at home or in social situations with your extended family and friends. How many hours a day do you lose on social media? What are you posting about yourself? Which image are you conveying, or trying to convey, in order to gain a few extra "likes" or thumbs-up? How crushing does it feel when it backfires and someone makes a comment that you consider rude or insulting?

Now, that's what I call hard work!

Many of my clients have a second addiction that they aren't even fully aware of and haven't come to me about – and that is their dependence on social media for recognition and approval. I see how reluctant they are to switch off their devices during our sessions, and how eager to reconnect as soon as our time together is over.

Some of them show me their pages proudly, with image after image of themselves in some seductive or contrived pose. They are almost always photos of shiny, happy people leading wonderful lives, yet the person showing me those photos may have just spent the previous hour in floods of tears telling me how unhappy they are.

This compulsion to depict their lives as perfect goes right to the heart of these clients' insecurities about themselves and the overwhelming need to be liked. It is also an example of what is known as "impostor syndrome" (see below).

Impostor Syndrome

Those with impostor syndrome continually question whether people like them and worry about their ability to perform the duties for which they were chosen. They generally remain deaf to any compliments about their success. Often perfectionists with a poor self-image, they will adopt a more discreet profile and evolve to a level of performance below their real capabilities. They cannot bring themselves to believe that they deserve the recognition they receive, and fear that one day they will be unmasked.

People with impostor syndrome often believe that it is just due to luck or good timing when they have achieved something at work or in their personal life. They have such a deep fear of being exposed for who they truly are, or as a "fraud", that they create an "impostor" persona – a kind of perfect avatar of themselves – in which they lead lives where they are always happy, where life is one big party, and where they are never plagued by anxiety or have to struggle like the rest of us.

I know of people who have paid for thousands of fake followers on social media just to look good, and others who immediately drop any "friends" if they start to complain about their lives in any way that is regarded as negative or imperfect. It is true that people who constantly moan – in person or online – can be toxic, but if social media allows us to constantly judge their comments or prune them out, then the only comparisons we allow ourselves with our own lives are wholly unrealistic ones. It also means that the only people we have to compare ourselves with appear to be good-looking, successful and happy (when they may well not be any of those things), which means that we can't possibly compete and will always be dissatisfied.

There will always be people who are better than you – whether they are more clever or more wealthy, have had greater success financially or in other ways, or have more children, bigger houses, nicer clothes, more luxurious holidays or better cars. Despite all that, we have no idea how they really feel deep down inside or what demons of their own they might be facing. We can never compete with them on all these levels, so why even try? There is only one you and your life is totally unique, so the only person you can compare yourself to is you.

Imagine how different life would be if we deliberately chose friends on social media who were far worse off than ourselves – people who were refugees or homeless, people in abusive relationships or with serious health problems. How about those with mental health issues, or the elderly and infirm suffering from chronic loneliness? If we compared ourselves to these "friends" instead, imagine how lucky we would feel – blessed in life and in good health. Their genuine problems would probably make our anxieties about carrying a little extra weight feel trivial and vain. Their misfortunes might inspire us to help them or do some good for those like them. What a different world it would be.

> "Social media gives me the chance to show off the best aspects of myself. I want all those people I went to school with to know that I made something of my life and that it worked out for me. Everyone knows that it's all for show anyway, but at least they can see that I have a lovely wife and a nice house and that I'm not the loser they thought I'd be."

Another client told me recently that her fake persona on social media backfired on her when – without her knowledge – friends booked a holiday she had gone on with her boyfriend that she had portrayed glowingly online. When the reality turned out to be far from perfect, the friends were horrified and publicly accused her of lying.

Many of my clients – especially the younger ones – spend hours online each day, deciding what photos to post that day and what to say about them. They doctor the pictures so that they look their best and then spend the rest of the day checking and rechecking to see how many people liked or commented on their post. A good "hit count" can make their day, whereas a poor one – or an adverse comment – can ruin it. And this from people they often don't even know personally. It takes so much energy and time, which they could be putting to better use in being mindful about their own way of life and eating habits. That's a much healthier pastime.

The crux of the matter here is self-confidence. Once we are comfortable in our own skin, and happy with our bodies and our lives, we no longer feel this constant need to seek approval. Clients often ask me if I think they should give up social media if it can be so detrimental to their self-confidence. I tell them, "Only if you want to. Maybe take a break from it for a while and see how that feels, but make sure you have a plan for what to do with the time you are freeing up, or you may find yourself eating more out of boredom." The decision should be yours once you have a better appreciation for yourself and do not want to compare your life to other people's all the time.

Many people who are overweight suffer from impostor syndrome in some form or other. They contrive to show a different aspect of themselves to compensate for what they see as the shameful, guilty secret of their unhealthy eating. The message might be, "I may be fat but, look, I'm fun and I know how to have a good time!"

Remember that I ask all my clients, "What is your secret that affects your self-worth?" Well, the answer is extremely relevant to this chapter. Many think their secret is that they have been deceiving people all along into thinking they are always good, always happy and always kind, when secretly they often feel mean, selfish and unhappy.

When I tell them that nobody is good all the time, and that we are all mean and selfish and unhappy sometimes, they discount that as some sort of trick. They cannot easily accept that all of us have a secret inner life in which we can be insecure and full of anxieties and worried about what others think of us too.

Sometimes the extra weight you carry can be a kind of signal to those around you that things aren't really that easy for you. It acts as a kind of red flag to wave to those who have fallen for the impostor persona to let them know that your life isn't quite as perfect as it seems. "I may be a high-achieving businesswoman, a mother and run a home as well, but – look – I can't even control my eating so don't expect too much of me."

Much of this often stems back to childhood and the way we were raised. If we had a "perfect" sibling who we were always compared to, or if nothing we ever did was quite good enough, then this can affect our self-confidence for years after, putting us in the ego state of the Child who is constantly seeking the approval of the Parent. Once we are grown, that "Parent" becomes the unknown "friends" on social media, or the boss at work, or the real friend who appears to have done better in life. It isn't healthy to judge your own life through the prism of someone else's.

If you think this applies to you, then try the following exercise to see if it makes you feel better about the real you and helps you to free yourself from the fake persona you have created to gain others' approval. Consider the questions and write down your answers if it helps.

- Did you receive adequate approval from your parents as a child?

- Was nothing you did ever good enough?

- Do you struggle sometimes with keeping up appearances for others?

- Do you feel as if you have failed in some way? If so, how?

- Are you always striving for perfection?

The thing to remember is that our real persona is not a million miles from the fake persona we project. Nobody can be good all the time. That would be frightening. We are each doing the best we can. That is all we can do. Some days we may do better than others, and when we have bad days we can hopefully learn from our mistakes, using the psychological or practical tools we need to achieve that goal. We are no different from anyone else, but what we may need to learn to do is to respect ourselves for who we are and what we have achieved. Unless we do this, guilt will only reinforce our sense of failure.

If we stop looking at others' lives for comparisons and remind ourselves of all that we have done – at work, at home, in relationships, as children, friends, siblings and parents – then we can stand tall with far more confidence and be proud of who we are. Any comparisons we make should be with who we were five years ago, not with someone we hardly know today.

I often tell my clients to take their right hand and place it on their left shoulder before patting themselves warmly in congratulation for getting this far. Self-respect has to start with us, long before we seek the respect and approval of others.

> **"In my family, everyone is overweight and always has been. If I start to lose weight, they will all feel like I am judging them in some way; that I think I'm better than they are. They will think that I am breaking away."**

Family networks can be the hardest to deal with when it comes to losing weight, especially within certain cultural groups. If most people in your family are overweight, you may be tempted to think that this is out of your control, that it's how things are supposed to be. "It's genetic," clients often tell me confidently. "I take after my father/mother. We have a long line of obesity in our family."

It doesn't take long to help them see that the reason they are overweight can be found not in their DNA but in their eating habits. The hardest part comes in dealing with the attitudes and opinions of the rest of the family when you step outside that cycle of overeating. Family members may find your independence confrontational. They may feel abandoned and regard you as no longer part of their group. Or at least this is what you may fear will happen.

In cases like this, we then have a decision to make. Do we want to keep the extra pounds in order to protect those we love even if it's at the expense of our happiness and health, or do we think it's legitimate to live the life we deserve?

One client told me he was dreading the weekly family get-together at his widowed mother's house. "She cooks for it all week and always makes far too much, so she sends us home with the leftovers. If we don't finish our plates, she takes it as a personal insult. I have made excuses not to go lately because I dread the temptation of all that food, and I don't want to upset her by not eating everything."

I countered by asking him, "But isn't she upset when you don't turn up? Would she feel worse not to see you at these happy family occasions, or to see you there fit and well and making the right choices about your life?"

If you find yourself in a situation like that, then I suggest that you speak privately to those you worry about offending or upsetting and gently ask how they feel and what they might be able to do to help you. This they can do by not being so intrusive or judgmental. They probably haven't even realized that their behaviour has impinged on your confidence or affected your resolve in any way and – if they really love you – they will be only too happy to do whatever they can to help you on your chosen path to happiness.

Here are some of the things you might say:

- I'm worried about the health implications of carrying this extra weight.

- I want to lose it so that I can live longer and in better health.

- I love what you cook for me but I'll no longer be eating so much of it.

- It would be great if you could help me with this.

- My decision to eat more healthily is deeply personal and I'm in no way rejecting or criticizing your own eating habits.

Similarly, in a family unit I suggest that people speak to their partners and their children to ask for understanding and respect in the choices they are making. By talking to those we are close to and sharing how we are feeling, we can open up a whole new dialogue that can be helpful and enlightening. Communication can be key – but remember, this is still your choice, your decision, and you don't want to obsess about it in an unhealthy way.

If you do feel that it would help to bring the subject up, go back in your mind to projecting yourself in the future and imagining yourself slim and fit, healthy and happy within your family gatherings. Think how that would feel and how differently you would behave. Think how those you love would treat you. If you feel it would be helpful to have a debate, ask your partners or children, "How do you feel about me having an issue with my body image? Would you be pleased if I lost weight? How would it be if I stopped talking about my weight so much?"

The responses will almost always be positive, which will give you more confidence to carry on with your journey to good health.

The reality is that even if it feels difficult at first to break away from the less healthy eating patterns of those around you, it's possible to have a positive impact on your network of friends and family by showing them that things can be different. They won't love you less, but you may well take a different place among them and maybe even be inspirational.

The truth is that most people don't care if their friend or wife or husband is carrying a few extra pounds. What they care about is how insecure or obsessed we are becoming when they hear it every day and have to repeatedly endure our suffering. Those in our networks are fed up with all the complaining and want it to end, as they can't do anything to help. Once we realize this, then we can stop obsessing unhealthily about others' opinions and judgments and start focusing on ourselves.

For those of us who have children, we can set a good example for their future by breaking this family pattern, and free them from the anxiety surrounding our health and body image.

> **"I was always so together and organized. I planned on being the best mother in the world but instead I put on a ton of weight, lost all my confidence, and ended up producing two grumpy teenagers who are as unhappy about their body shape as I am about mine. I feel such a failure."**

Unless we address our own weight issues, once we have children we can inadvertently pass on our bad habits to our offspring. We don't mean to, but we may well have lost our own intuition and spontaneity. All it often takes is a little self-reflection on what effect our parents' behaviour may have had on us.

For example, if we were consistently told to "finish your plate" and punished if we didn't (as I was), then that can continue into adulthood in the psyche and set a deep-rooted pattern of eating long after we are sated. If we then force our own child to empty the plate and even congratulate him or her afterward, we are creating the same kind of pattern, one that they will struggle to get rid of as adults.

I don't blame anyone for doing this because, of course, we all want our children to eat well and enjoy the food that we have lovingly prepared. It is hard to accept that our child may be in a better place than we are to know when he or she has had enough. Children often want to stop eating because they know there is dessert, which they're usually keener on than other food. That's why I recommend several rules for meals:

- There shouldn't be a dessert after every meal. Why accustom your child to always finish their dinner with something sweet? If you do want to offer a dessert, serve it later on so that they don't get used to eating too quickly in order to get to it.

- Never rush your child when eating, even if it can be boring waiting for them to finish. You don't have to sit by their side throughout – you can do your own thing and come back to the table from time to time. Try not to have too much distraction while your child is eating either. Music is fine, but please avoid the television and/or video games. Ask your child what they think about the food – how it tastes and the texture – and listen to their responses non-judgmentally, without making them feel guilty if they are less than enthusiastic. The idea is to make them more mindful about eating from an early age, in order to develop that skill.

■ Encourage your children to become involved in the preparation and cooking of food from an early age, even if it is just washing or chopping the vegetables. They'll soon become more familiar with all the ingredients instead of just seeing a plate land in front of them. Share your enthusiasm for food too, telling them what your favourite things are and how you like them cooked.

■ If you have more than one child, please don't make comparisons between them such as, "See, your sister is finished already," or, "But your brother really likes it, so why don't you?" Everyone is different in terms of taste and the pace at which they eat – and should be respected for that.

■ Try not to use food as a reward – giving your child chocolate when he or she is crying or upset could set a pattern that they are stuck with for life. Instead, comfort them and talk to them about why they're upset. It may take longer than the chocolate, but it is so much healthier psychologically!

■ Parents often complain that their kids will automatically reach for sweets and won't eat fruit. Find out which fruit your child prefers and offer them more than one option. Make fruit easily accessible, far more than sweets. Smoothies and fresh fruit juices are good in small quantities too, but keep in mind that these contain more sugar and less fibre than whole fruits.

■ It isn't helpful to tell children that certain foods like pizza or burgers are "bad" or taboo. Instead, explain that they aren't the healthiest options and should be eaten only once in a while.

One problem that concerns me deeply is the impact on children of a parent who is unhappy about their body shape and weight and talks continuously about it. Kids who have been forced to live with the food anxieties of adults throughout their childhood will often start to mimic these bad habits and may be headed for a similar lifetime of obsession – thus continuing the unhappy cycle.

It doesn't have to be like this.

There is another way.

In the best-case scenario the child will see how toxic it is to be obsessed with food or weight and won't act in the same way, but more often than not they will inherit these unhealthy compulsions and become overly body conscious and worried about their weight from an alarmingly tender age. It's okay to explain to your children that you're not happy with certain things about yourself, but it shouldn't invade their territory hourly, every day or even at every meal. If it does, the weight issue will quickly take up far too much room in the relationship and create a distance between you and your child.

Another issue is when one child grows up to be heavier than another. This can present problems too, especially if the parents compare the child to his or her thinner siblings. "You must take after your father, Jack. His whole family is fat. Thank God, your sister takes after me." In the interest of all your children, comparisons like these should never be made. Far from helping or motivating the child, it will make them even more self-conscious and never allow them to understand that we are all very different in this highly personal matter.

I know this is a lot to take in, but it is often only when you realize that you have done some of these things that you can make changes and behave differently with your children. Think of it as a wake-up call to make lasting improvements in their lives, and yours.

TO RECAP

- Family patterns can affect our weight – if everyone in your family is overweight, then it's scary being the one to lose weight first. It can feel as if we are leaving the rest of our family behind. The same goes for friends.

- Cultural influences have a similar effect. In some groups, to be overweight is not only acceptable but desirable and people only feel different or uncomfortable with their bodies when they're at work or parted from their "tribe".

- Peer group pressure can be another negative influence – accept that to stay in that overweight "impostor persona" you have adopted, you may be trying to feel less threatening in some way or because you want to be the reliable, comfortable, happy one.

- Avoid comparing yourself with others. See social media for what it is and engage only if you are able to detach yourself from others' lives and not compare them to your own. You have plenty of your own issues to deal with mindfully without wasting hours fretting about your so-called friends.

- Give yourself more credit – learn to appreciate that everyone has their own struggles and anxieties just like you, as well as an inner secret life. Accept that you have done the best you can and make plans to do even better in the future.

- Respect yourself – remind yourself of all that you have achieved and look at your life in Adult mode, not as the judgmental Parent or the needy Child. The best recognition is that you give to yourself.

CASE STUDY

Paul is a 47-year-old hedge fund manager who has a seemingly beautiful life, but he is deeply unhappy because his weight has ballooned to 115 kilos (18 stone).

He is far from a child, but he and his wife have developed a Child/Parent relationship in which she mothers him, which means that he will mostly respond in Child mode. "Why are you eating cake again?" she might challenge him, and he'll feel guilty but finish it anyway, allowing his rebellious Child to respond. Or she'll serve him a full plate of food when he isn't that hungry because he ate a snack at 4pm. If he explained this to her and asked to serve himself according to his needs, then he would probably eat what he needed to. But the child in him responds to the mother in her that sees her role as a homemaker, cook and parent, so he eats the meal to please her or, at least, not disappoint her.

It is a game but, as in most games, if one player stops taking part then the game stops by itself and leaves the other player high and dry.

This kind of role-play may have first come about because Paul complains about his weight all the time to his wife, friends and family, and feels that this has become their chief topic of conversation. By speaking about his weight so often, Paul doesn't face his responsibility in overeating, he is only reinforcing a negative image of himself and sharing his anxiety with his wife. When he constantly tells people that he feels fat or wishes he hasn't eaten so much, he is giving them responsibility that they don't possess. They are helpless to do anything about his weight and they're tired of hearing him complain.

I suggested to Paul that he stop talking about his weight and food intake in any way for a week or more and was able to help him see that this was a much bigger problem in his mind than it was in the minds of those he lived with. The people around him loved him regardless of his size or shape and just wanted him to be happy and free of his constant anxiety about his appearance.

When he stopped talking endlessly about his weight, it gave him and his wife room to share other things and remove a lot of stress from their relationship. This freed him to regain full responsibility for what he was eating and how much. It is often tempting to fall back into bad patterns to fill the gaps we may have in our relationships, but these are gaps that we must learn to live with or whose relevance and meaning we must at least try to understand.

5

EAT MORE MINDFULLY, POSITIVELY AND INTUITIVELY

"When I was a kid we used to sit around the dinner table as a family and take an hour over our meal, chatting about our day. Now my family all seem to eat on the run, bolting down a few mouthfuls before heading back out the door."

This chapter introduces the Food and Emotions Diary, which is the most important tool in my therapy toolkit. The diary is the best way of seeing what, when and how you are eating, and also to understand the tricks your emotions are playing on you.

You will learn how to differentiate the signals your body sends you when it needs food from the ones that come from your emotional brain. At last you will be able to eat according to your hunger and satiety and respond healthily to your needs.

Eating mindfully will help you eat quantities that match your hunger, in a way that is pleasurable and at the right pace. Eating positively will allow you to focus on what to eat instead of what not to eat. You will then stop being scared by certain types of food. Eating intuitively means that you will listen to your body's needs in terms of energy, nutrients and variety. Some people convince themselves they have a food addiction, which only reinforces the idea that there is not much they can do about their eating.

In fact, many different things influence the way we eat – factors that we may not even be fully aware of:

- **Where we are** – in a restaurant, at home, while walking, at work or commuting. Do we have a free hand for the food we are eating? Can we easily leave it or take it home if we don't finish it? Are others watching us eat? Will we eat quickly when we're sat on the sofa because we're worried about leaving a stain?

- **What we're doing** while eating – playing a game, reading the news, chatting online, browsing social networks, watching television, or shopping online. Clients who buy things on auction sites tell me the stress of the auction often makes them snack more. Others find watching sports usually leads to drinking too much and eating too many unhealthy snacks.

- **Who we're with** – a friend or group of friends, our partner, alone, with our kids, with colleagues or at a business dinner. We may eat lightly in company, not wanting to be seen to overeat for fear of being judged, then binge eat when we are home. Or our companions may urge us to match their intake of food and drink, or expect us to eat like for like if we are in a business situation.

- **What our posture is** – lying in bed, standing on a train or at a bar, slouching on a sofa or sitting at a table hunched over our plates. Are we able to sit comfortably, breathe freely, and give ourselves the physical and emotional distance we need before we begin to eat our food?

- **How stressed or pressured we feel** – stress is very common among overeaters who feel that they never have enough time, and are constantly exhausted through lack of sleep or anxiety. They seek sweet, sugary things to raise their blood sugar and give them a quick "fix".

We tend not to see how these things can impact our eating patterns, or realize how they can have a negative effect on our weight. This is because we are often not being mindful enough about what we are eating and why, and may just be consuming calories because that's what we've planned to do or what others around us are doing.

In several of these situations, in which conditions, cues, social norms and acquired habits often lead us to food, it's quite hard to know how hungry we really are and to accurately gauge when we are full. We may always consume popcorn and chocolates when we go to the movies, for example, eat fries every Friday, or traditionally finish a meal with an ice cream regardless of whether we want it or not.

When I was first divorced and I had my children to stay every two weeks, I worked hard to make sure everything was perfect for their visit, preparing good food and eating it with them. I wanted to be the ideal father, so I never invited friends and always gave the children my fullest attention. But when the kids went to bed, I was on my own with no one to talk to and all the leftovers, which I often ate out of boredom or loneliness. A friend of mine suggested I invite people over sometimes to help entertain my kids and to keep me company after their bedtime. It worked. The kids enjoyed the livelier atmosphere and I didn't eat for comfort on my own.

The sense of being pressured by time is a huge factor too. Many of us eat the way we live, which most often is hectically. If we grab something "on the run", then we are not tuning in to what our body is telling us we should eat or appreciate whether or not we are eating at a healthy pace. This complete detachment from what we are putting into our mouths is very common and extremely dangerous for those who have a tendency to overeat. Many of the clients I start working with can't even remember what they ate at their last meal; for them it was simply a question of refuelling on autopilot.

> "When I come in from work I only have half an hour before meeting my friends down the pub so it's easier to buy a takeaway or heat a pizza quickly in the microwave. The trouble is, I'm now doing that five nights a week."

Most of us tend to eat and drink far too quickly, never allowing ourselves the minimum ten to fifteen minutes it takes for the stomach to alert the brain that it is full. By that time we'll have probably finished our plate (and maybe even had a second helping) and moved on to busying ourselves with something else. Throughout my careers as both restaurateur and psychotherapist, I have rarely seen slow eaters who are overweight.

Our body is an amazing machine, full of sensors that send us all kinds of signals all day long, and yet we lead such busy lives that we tend not to listen to these as much as we should anymore. Each time we put something in our mouths, thousands of tiny receptors assess the food for taste and texture and allow us to decide if it is salty or sweet, tasty or not. If it meets with our approval, we chew it and swallow it, followed quickly by the next mouthful and so on until the plate is empty.

It isn't until the food has been processed in this way and passed down the oesophagus and into the stomach, though, that the gut begins to absorb the glucose and other nutrients and release the satiety hormones that travel to the brain to let us know that we have had enough. This "disconnect" is what allows us to keep eating more than we need to before we have even realized that we're full.

"Go on, you can have just one more," is a common thought my clients tell me they have at the end of a meal, along with, "I could hardly move afterward, I ate so much!"

Mindfulness

Mindfulness is the process of focusing one's attention on the present on a moment-to-moment basis. Originating in Eastern practices of meditation and Buddhism, it is a way of paying special attention to what you are doing right now, with special focus on the breathing. This is done to develop self-awareness and to free the mind of anxiety, depression and stress. By concentrating on "the now" we are able to push all other thoughts aside and calmly appreciate what we are doing in a way that leads to a positive mental state.

True mindfulness (see above), especially mindful eating, is not an easy thing to accomplish, even though it is an interesting practice with fascinating results. It is certainly worth squeezing it into our everyday lives as a deliberate choice. My clients so often tell me that they are "too busy to be mindful" and talk about how little spare time they have as if it is out of their control, but all that's happening is that they are not taking responsibility for their own actions and decisions. It's a question of time management and keeping some time for yourself. Besides, eating an everyday meal only takes a matter of minutes, so we can easily afford to take a few more. This is not a radical change.

Even though we might think we don't have the time to be mindful, we can easily adapt the technique to our own circumstances. And when we read about its benefits the question we have to ask ourselves is, can we afford not to be mindful? People who are able to practise mindfulness properly are not only found to live longer and more healthily, but they are generally happier, have better careers and relationships, and are even better able to defend themselves against disease.

Yet, so many of us don't take full advantage of this free daily tool that could have a dramatic impact on every aspect of our lives. We don't choose to eat the food that we know we should. We don't stop eating when we've had enough. We don't turn everything off and take a break when we feel tired. We don't stay away from the people who have a negative impact on us, and so on.

Few of us live the lives of Buddhist monks or can afford to spend long periods of time contemplating life in all its minutiae: watching, smelling or caressing the food we're about to eat. It's not possible to ask everyone in a café or restaurant to be silent while we're eating so that we can concentrate on all the sensations. Not many of us seem to be able to find the time to meditate daily. Yet because we don't do these things and consequently feel so pressured and lost, we often turn our attention instead to "gurus" and self-help authors in the quest for quick solutions or instant remedies. We can surely be inspired by some of these people, but in the end we are all different and need to find our own way to get the best out of life.

> **I have spent a small fortune on diet cookbooks as well as happiness guides and books about Danish 'hygge', but none of it works for long. I would have been better off giving the money to charity and spending the time doing some deep breathing and simple mindfulness, which finally made a difference.**

I believe there is a balance to be found between "extreme" mindful eating and what has become "mind-less" eating, so that we can enjoy our meals in a way in which we are much more connected with our senses and more aware of our needs. Each of us can realistically adopt new habits that will enable us to stop eating when we're full, instead of constantly feeling that we have guzzled our food too quickly or eaten too much.

Only when we are tuned in to the information our body is sending us can we eat much more healthily. Unfortunately, many things can get in the way and make this difficult or even impossible:

- **Processed foods** such as ready-made lasagnes, pizzas or meat pies often contain so much fat, salt and hidden sugar that our taste buds can be altered if we consume too much of them. This means that we are no longer tempted by fresh fruit and vegetables, as without all that extra flavouring they don't seem so tasty. We all know that we should only eat processed foods occasionally, but they are quick, easy and convenient, and – with time and repetition – can become addictive.

- **Tiredness** has a huge influence on our food choices too, as we tend to choose food that will provide us with a quick energy fix. The problem is that sugary snacks make our glycaemic index rise and fall very quickly, leaving us with a feeling of hunger. Being tired also makes us more inclined to be moody and therefore choose comfort food.

- **Alcohol** will easily distract us from our feeling of satiety and often makes us choose more calorific food, as it contains higher quantities of sugar. When we are drinking, our sense of responsibility diminishes, and we feel the urge to "have fun" and forget about being healthy or good. And when we are hungover, the tendency is to reach for rich, fatty foods to take the edge off. There will be more about this in Chapter 8.

- **Our emotions,** when not taken into account appropriately, will have a huge influence on our food choices and quantities, as discussed in previous chapters. Thinking about what we are next going to eat – whether it be a snack or a meal – can distract us from other thoughts. Thoughts about food pop into our mind with a connected internal dialogue such as:

"I'd like to eat something."
"Oh, but I shouldn't as I ate something not so long ago."
"Yes, but I really feel like it."

"What am I going to eat, then?"
"No, I shouldn't have that, it's fattening."
"Yes, but it'll be okay if I don't eat later on."

Then afterward:

"Why did I eat all that? I don't feel good."
"I'm useless and I'll always be fat…"

All these kinds of thoughts can keep us busy for several minutes at a time!

Whenever we overeat, we are anaesthetizing the emotions that are too difficult to deal with. Having food as a distraction can achieve this, but never for long as – before we know it – we're confronted with them again. And each time we succumb to cravings, our confidence takes a knock and we tend to need to eat even more.

Emotions that aren't properly dealt with don't disappear, unfortunately, and all we are doing is piling more on, one on top of the other. This lack of respect for what and how we feel plays tricks on us. We can put our emotions aside only if we do it in a conscious way. Say, for example, someone has spoken disrespectfully to you at work. You can decide to defer your response to a time that suits you. You can say to yourself, "I didn't like the way that person talked to me and I will deal with that when we meet again later today, but at the moment I have to attend this meeting and I don't want that feeling to interfere." Once again, being in tune with how we feel and why we feel this way will allow us to make the necessary changes in order not to overeat to compensate.

▨ **Peer group pressure** – we have already discussed the effect of those around us but it is also relevant here, when it comes to the daily influences I will ask you to think about when filling in your Food and Emotions Diary.

You may think at first that there are too many things to take into account when eating, and you'd be right, but that's because they all have an influence on us and can interfere with our wellbeing. Instead of feeling as if you have to control all these elements, consider it more like a spring-clean of your mind, sifting the debris room by room. I will help you sort out things that consume so much of your energy and time without you even realizing it.

Start by filling in the Food and Emotions Diary (see opposite) every day, for a couple of weeks at least. It shouldn't take you more than a few minutes each day. The important thing is for you to enter the data before and during every meal, so that you are fully in the moment and haven't had time to embellish or forget. This will also allow you to pause, lean back, take a breath, and really consider what you are about to consume before you even begin to eat. I recommend this to all my clients, along with taking a few pauses during every meal. Put down your cutlery, breathe, think about how hungry you are and take a few seconds to look at the food in front of you to assess how much more you will need to consume.

By taking the time to think about these important questions and writing down your answers, you will really have to think about what you're doing. If you forget to fill in the diary at some point, it's all right – just get back to it the next time you're about to eat.

The main aim of this precious tool is to get you to be more mindful when you're eating, by separating your body sensations (hunger and satiety) from your emotions.

"Every time I eat I finish everything on my plate because I don't want to waste anything, especially if I've paid for it."

Below is a blank diary, seven copies of which – one for each day of the week – are provided at the back of this book (see pages 242–55). You can also download it from my website to print out and fill in (see page 265). Alternatively, you can set it up yourself on your computer, phone or tablet – whatever best works for you.

The idea is to have your diary quickly and easily to hand and to get into the habit of filling it in at every meal or snack. It doesn't take long to do, and once you do get into the habit you will come to think of it as a normal part of your eating experience.

Day	Food and Drinks	Emotions and Context	Hunger/Satiety/Pleasure
Morning			
Noon			
Afternoon			
Evening			

As you can see, the diary is divided into a grid system with four horizontal columns for morning, noon, afternoon and evening, with three vertical sections representing food and drink, emotions and context, hunger/satiety and pleasure. Those of you who snack in the night should add an additional column.

Let's take a closer look at the kinds of things I would like you to insert in the blank spaces:

DAY

This is obvious. You simply enter the day of the week and the date. The reason for this is that you will quite rapidly see if there is a pattern which emerges on certain days of the week. Some people eat quite healthily during the week but will indulge themselves during the weekend, for example. Others will tend to overeat mostly in the evening. Many will find it more difficult to be mindful on the days or weeks when their children are with them. Holidays and travel can make things more complicated for some of us. We will first find out what the pattern is and then see how you can fix the issues.

FOOD AND DRINKS

This is the place to list the food you are having, so you might be eating a ham and cheese sandwich on white bread with extra mayonnaise, a kebab, or maybe a slice of pie. You don't need to weigh it or write down the specific ingredients, but I would like you to estimate the size of what you're about to eat, for example "a small bowl of granola", or "a large plate of pasta with quite a lot of grated cheese" or "a generous wedge of cake". You need only write down drinks such as soft drinks including fruit juices, coffee or tea with milk and/or sugar, and alcohol. Be sure not to miss anything out, like the little chocolate biscuit or cookie that sometimes comes on the saucer of your coffee.

EMOTIONS AND CONTEXT

This is the place to enter how you feel when you're about to have that meal. Try to identify which emotion you're experiencing. Are you perhaps angry with someone at work, or upset by something a friend or partner said? Do you feel happy because the sun is shining, or sad because you are facing family difficulties? Are you worried about money, your job, your kids? If you find it difficult to identify an emotion, ask yourself what you are thinking about in that moment and this might help you realize which emotion it brings up. Our brain is always active and I would like you to see if you can sort those thoughts for a moment. We have seen in earlier chapters how to address the messages that our emotions are sending us.

As for context, here is where I want you to write where you are and with whom when you eat. For example, *Eating by myself in front of the computer*, or *Grabbing a quick sandwich on my commuter train*, *Watching TV with my kids*, or *At a business dinner with clients*.

The idea is to separate what you feel in terms of hunger from what your mind is telling you in terms of your emotions. You might write, *I'm in a café with a friend who is whining about their problems. I feel tired and stressed.* Or, *I'm embarrassed because I'm on a busy train eating a sausage roll quickly so people don't stare at me. I'll have to eat it all or I'll have the rest dropping crumbs everywhere*, or, *I am angry that I'm eating and drinking more than I need because I'm with a client who's ordered all three courses and some wine and I don't want to offend her.*

Connecting to our emotions is not an easy thing at first, so be patient with the process as it could take time and practice. You might not feel like doing it sometimes if you fear it could be overwhelming, and I understand that, but remember that finding out which emotions you're dealing with will not make you more vulnerable.

HUNGER/SATIETY/PLEASURE

It is important to think about and then write down how hungry you are before you start eating. Look at the food in front of you for a moment and decide if you really are hungry enough to finish it all. It's fine if you are, but if you're chiefly eating because it is your designated lunch break, or because someone has prepared it for you, I would like you to take that into account.

I would also like you to think about your hunger again after the first course or at the halfway point of the meal. Are you still hungry? Do you need to finish the plate? Is this enough or will you choose something as a second course? Remember that this may change while you're eating, so estimate your hunger at the beginning and then see how you feel.

Then write down how sated and satisfied you feel when you've finished eating your meal. Do you feel as if you have overeaten? The same goes for pleasure. Are you enjoying what you're having? Do you keep on enjoying it in the same way when you've eaten half of it? This is also valid for your drinks.

Here are two examples of diaries kept by people I have called Sophie and Robert, showing the changes in their eating choices over the four weeks. These will be the two case studies for this chapter.

SOPHIE

Sophie is a bubbly 36-year-old who lives and works in London. She has been single for two years and she is employed by a media company as a creative. She doesn't have children and she is fine with that. She has put on about 12 kilos (2 stone) in the last 18 months even though she's relatively active physically.

She finds it very difficult to say no to others, as she fears that they won't like her if she does. She puts herself under a lot of pressure and is working for a company that is reducing its staff, which doesn't help, even though her own job is not at stake.

Her over-empathy means that her colleagues' stress becomes hers: she doesn't have clear enough boundaries between their lives and her own. To make matters worse, for various reasons she has been socializing with friends less and less over the years and often feels quite lonely.

On the upside, in general she's not unhappy about her life as there are many good things about it - she likes working as a creative, she is in good health, she's doing quite well financially, she loves the flat she bought a few years ago, and she enjoys going for a run a few times a week.

SOPHIE'S DIARY, WEEK 1

Day TUESDAY	Food and Drinks	Emotions and Context	Hunger/Satiety/Pleasure
Morning	7am Porridge/ skimmed milk Medium bowl Coffee (black)	Sleepy and in a hurry, long day ahead.	I don't know if I'm hungry but I feel I have to eat. I've loved porridge since I was little.
	At 11, half Cheddar sandwich (bought it on my way to the office)	Angry and stressed, huge pressure in my department!!! Eating at my desk between two meetings.	Hungry, I pause when I'm done with the first half and stop as not hungry anymore: yes! ;) I really enjoy it.
Noon	1pm other half Cheddar sandwich Black tea	Exhausted, bored, empty... In the office kitchen, standing with other colleagues sharing their stress.	Not really hungry but everyone is having a lunch break. I enjoy it less than earlier.
	Two portions of birthday cake...	I couldn't say no as the cake was prepared by one of my colleagues and she's obviously very proud of her mother's recipe. I realize I'm irritated by how pushy she is with things.	Didn't like it and felt like I was having a sugar attack afterward!!
Afternoon	4.30pm apple	On my way to the station, glad I'm done with work.	Very hungry before and still hungry when I'm done. Love those Granny Smith apples!!!
Evening	8pm 2 large glasses of wine, roasted nuts	In my neighbour's garden, relaxing at last.	Very hungry but we've planned to go out for dinner so I'll manage with nuts. Enjoying the wine.
	8.45pm Fish & chips About half a bottle of wine & a G&T (slimline)	At our local pub with my neighbour, happy & tipsy.	Hungry when I start, ate all the plate but should have stopped earlier as I feel it was too much. Ate far too quickly... Had the wine to join the others but didn't really enjoy.
	11pm Small bag of M&M's	Tired, in bed watching TV, lonely again...	Not hungry (obviously!!!) but feel like having a treat.

SOPHIE'S DIARY, WEEK 4

Day TUESDAY	Food and Drinks	Emotions and Context	Hunger/Satiety/Pleasure
Morning	10am Porridge/skimmed milk Small portion	I take a 10 mins break in the office kitchen and eat at relaxed pace. I was worried this morning about a friend's health but I'm able to put these thoughts aside now as I've decided to pay her a visit this Saturday.	I start being hungry, sated afterward, really good
Noon	1pm Salad with falafels & beetroots at a nearby café	Decided to go out for lunch with my colleague Yolanda. It feels good to take some fresh air and walk a bit instead of staying in. Taking some time with her has made me realize we have a lot in common and I appreciate her. I guess I'm just feeling relaxed.	Quite hungry to start with, I paused at some point and noticed I was still hungry so finished it. I love that salad and I'll try to match their recipe at home.
Afternoon	5pm a tiny bit of hummus with carrot sticks I brought from home	Tired and a bit worried about the drink tonight for the school reunion. I want to make sure I won't drink or eat too much. I think I'll manage it well. I eat in front of my computer but I make sure I don't rush.	A bit hungry, a bit bland in fact...
	6pm apple	In the train.	My treat! Not hungry.
Evening	8pm Bresaola and mushroom A glass of cava Sea bass with fennel and 2 new potatoes ;) A glass of red wine	I'm actually more happy to be here than I thought I'd be. We're having fun! Some of them drink a lot of cava and/or wine and I'm glad I'm not. It doesn't stop me from being close to them and laughing. We're in an old-fashioned restaurant in the city centre but it doesn't matter much.	Hungry, I decide to take a light starter. I leave a bit of sea bass as I've had enough. Cava and wine were OK... Some of them order a pudding but I don't feel like it.

Let's take Sophie's diary and look at what and how she eats. In Week One, she has breakfast although she is not hungry yet. Although there is nothing wrong with eating porridge, why would you give your body food when it's clearly telling you it doesn't need any? She then eats half a sandwich at 11am. when she is next hungry. Knowing that she has to fill in her diary, she notices that she has had enough and leaves half of the sandwich.

At lunch, she eats the second half of her sandwich only in order to join in with the others. This gives legitimacy to the food she's having as she would feel "weird" if she was the only one there not eating. Owing in part to the tensions in her company, where she feels bad because some of the staff have been made redundant, she doesn't dare say no to the cake she's being offered. Sharing it makes her feel more a part of the team. Yet she's annoyed at her colleague who's insisting she should have another slice. It is obvious to me that she is really angry and frustrated by her incapacity to refuse. The colleague in this case reminds Sophie of her mother who was a feeder and would be happy only when everything she cooked had been eaten.

Later that afternoon she eats only an apple although she is very hungry. She thinks it's better not to eat anything else now because she knows she will indulge herself in the evening. It's funny to note how we unconsciously plan our unhealthy eating experiences.

Before dinner, she eats almonds to manage her growing hunger, although nuts may not be the healthiest option before a heavy dinner. When she is finally having her meal, she eats far too quickly because she's so hungry. She then feels bloated, and it's not unusual to feel that alcohol will diminish that sensation. And, because she feels bad physically as well as guilty, she believes that alcohol might alleviate those feelings and make her less self-conscious. Later at night she finds the chocolates comforting and then she tells herself that it doesn't matter anyway, because the day has been a failure.

By Week Four, Sophie has reached a better understanding of her own habits. She is having breakfast when she is hungry and as a consequence she is not hungry for the rest of the morning. She finds out which emotion she's dealing with and how to manage it so that she can can start eating more mindfully.

Having a proper lunch break helps her relax properly and connects her with someone who was in her perimeter but she hadn't previously noticed. She has a snack later on in the afternoon as she feels hungry and she knows that it will help her eat more healthily later on. We can see clearly here that she is planning to be more gentle with herself throughout the day. She is in a positive mindset, not a diet one.

By dinnertime, she is making healthy choices, choosing to have a starter so as not to be too hungry by the time the main dish is served. She can resist the dessert because she feels sated, she enjoyed what she ate and drank, and doesn't feel frustrated at all.

Sophie has now lost all the weight she wanted to. It took her about six months to achieve and she has been slim for three years. She sends me an email every once in a while to share her enthusiasm about the things she keeps on discovering about herself. She now works for another company which has much better vibes. Most of all, she is happy.

"If someone cries, then I cry too. If they laugh, then I can't help but join in. Taking on other people's emotions all the time is exhausting and makes me feel very drained. That's usually when I reach for the cookie tin or the chocolate drawer."

ROBERT

Robert is a very kind chap, too kind in fact, and he pays a price for this. He is a pleaser, making sure everybody around him is happy and that there is no tension among his friends and colleagues. On a daily basis he finds it very difficult to relax as he is pretty much in control all the time. He shares his life with his wife Gina and their three children and and they're a lovely family. Robert has a good business, having created his own spirit brand, which can now be found in the country's best bars and restaurants.

Within the last seven years he has put on 27 kilos (four and a half stone). The success of his business and the attention it requires makes him fearful that he won't take good enough care of his family and friends and at some point things might go wrong. He comes from a family for whom being happy and sociable means sharing food and drinks in large quantities. During our initial sessions I immediately told Robert that he had to stop feeling responsible for others. It was time to take care of himself.

He agreed to make some changes in his beliefs and his ways of doing certain things. He was still scared that his world would fall apart, but as we went through these fears in a calm and systematic way he realized that the people around him and the life he had were not nearly as fragile as he had feared.

ROBERT'S DIARY, WEEK 1

Day SUNDAY	Food and Drinks	Emotions and Context	Hunger/Satiety/Pleasure
Morning	10am 5 pancakes with maple syrup 2 large glasses of orange juice	I feel tired and hungover, ate and drank too much yesterday evening at the business dinner. I don't want to show my wife and kids that I'd rather be in bed with a book. I don't want to disappoint them and I feel like these family moments are precious.	Not hungry but I make pancakes for Gina and the kids: it's our Sunday ritual!
	11.30am a few slices of ham	By myself, relaxing in the garden.	A bit hungry, still hungry afterward
Noon	1pm a piece of toast with mature cheddar and a tomato	At the kitchen table, checking my emails to make sure I haven't left any behind (I know, it's Sunday!!!)	Quite hungry but I don't want to eat too much as we're having Sunday roast later on. Still hungry afterward
Afternoon	3pm Sunday roast: the Full Monty!! A pint of lager when we arrive as I was very thirsty. 3 more pints while we're there	With Gina and the kids at our local pub. Other friends join us and we'll watch the rugby. I'm stressed as I want to make sure everyone is having a good time. As more friends join us, I'm concerned they'll all appreciate each other... I feel very tired later – too much pressure, too much noise, not such a relaxing Sunday afternoon at the end.	Very very hungry, ate far too quickly and I feel really bad afterward as my stomach hurts. I think I've enjoyed the taste of it, at the beginning at least.
Evening	8.30pm 3 slices of pizza, leftovers from the kids' dinner, a glass of red wine	Watching television on the sofa with Gina, drained but happy as it feels like mission accomplished.	Can't remember to be honest but I guess not. Enjoyed it.
	9.30pm Another glass of red wine	My reward for being a good husband, parent, friend... And I like sharing this with Gina.	Enjoyed it.

ROBERT'S DIARY WEEK 4

Day SUNDAY	Food and Drinks	Emotions and Context	Hunger/Satiety/Pleasure
Morning	9.30am 2 scrambled eggs and a bit of smoked salmon	I feel rested, I didn't overeat or drink yesterday evening and I then slept much better. I'm looking forward to this day. By myself in the kitchen, reading the Sunday newspaper.	Kind of hungry, enjoyed it and glad I've cooked 2 eggs instead of the 3 I originally planned.
	10.30am 2 pancakes	I know I'll only have one next Sunday but I want to keep it as a tradition.	Not hungry, left half of the second pancake and the dog enjoyed the other half. Enjoyed it.
Noon	1.30pm Cherry tomatoes and mozzarella, basil Water!!	I eat at a relaxed pace in the kitchen with Gina. I feel slightly stressed that we haven't booked our holiday yet and decide I'll do this with Gina tomorrow evening.	Kind of hungry so I eat not to be starving by the time we get to the pub.
Afternoon	3pm Sunday roast, I decide to have the chicken. 2 medium glasses of red wine and loads of water (I now realize how thirsty I can get!!)	I have told friends that we would be at the pub. I didn't organize anything for us all to meet. I felt relieved that I didn't have to control anything: I don't want to be in charge anymore! We've had a very nice time until we felt like it was time to go and relax at home.	A bit hungry. I left a few roast potatoes on the side and didn't feel the need to finish the gravy. I really enjoyed it and feel full when I decide to stop. I go for a better wine to indulge myself.
Evening	7pm Dinner with the kids ;) Nice salade niçoise, green beans, potatoes, crunchy leaves, anchovies, tomatoes	We decide to eat in the garden as it is a warm evening. I feel relaxed, I wish tomorrow wasn't Monday but I manage to put that thought aside.	Hungry and loved it! Not hungry for a second serving.
	8pm A few cherries	In the garden, no particular feeling.	Not hungry, delicious!
	A small glass of red wine	With Gina on the sofa, watching TV	It's OUR moment!

Now let's take a look at Robert's diary. In Week One he ate five pancakes for breakfast, not because he was hungry but to please everyone, and to keep the tradition – as he says. He is hungover and tired, and this combination makes him feel as if he needs sugary food. He is also hungry later on and eats slices of ham and toast. His sugary breakfast hasn't left him with any sense of long-term fullness.

He is far too hungry by the time he starts his Sunday roast lunch, and therefore he eats far too quickly to acknowledge whether or not he is sated at any point. Like many people, Robert doesn't drink enough water – he is simply not used to it – so he'll have alcoholic drinks which dehydrate him even more. This means he'll order even more of them in an subconscious attempt to quench his thirst.

By dinner time he is not hungry, but his pizza and wine will comfort him and calm his frustration.

By Week Four, Robert starts his day more rested as he has been able to drink and eat reasonably the night before. He is hungry and chooses to eat something that he likes and that will make him feel fuller for longer. He eats one and a half pancakes as he is mindful enough to note that he doesn't feel like any more. He now knows how to pay more attention to his thirst all day long, which will prevent him from drinking too much alcohol that could, on top of escalating his calorie intake, make him feel tired and go for unhealthy food choices.

As lunchtime approaches, he notices he is hungry and decides to have a light snack before his Sunday roast so that he'll find it much easier to manage his food intake at the restaurant. He knows things get more difficult while he is there because he has quite a few friends around. He chooses healthier chicken instead of pork, and he is able to leave some food on the side. He is much more relaxed as he has made the decision to not be responsible for his friends. He notices that the event goes smoothly without him having to control everything. He told me he regretted all the energy he spent all those years for no reason.

"It's not time for regrets," I told him. "It's time to be delighted for what's ahead of you."

For dinner, Robert has a reasonable portion of a healthy salad and some red wine. Altogether he has eaten and drunk a lot less and has felt much better all day long. He doesn't feel any guilt for the wine he had, nor did he this morning for the pancakes. This makes him feel better about himself generally.

Robert lost his first 6 kilos (1 stone) within the first four weeks and five months later he was back to his healthy weight. I can hear you shouting at me: "Five months? That's a lifetime!" I know you want instant results – a miracle that will make you slim and look younger in just a few days – but be sensible.

During these six months Robert has felt better day after day. He is more rested, less stressed, feels more mindful and connected to the people that he cares for, and in a more spontaneous way. The six months haven't at all been about dieting for him; they have been about his needs and how he is now writing this exciting next chapter of his life.

"I used to complain that it wasn't fair that I was fat because I ate pretty healthily. It was only when I really paid attention to how much I put in my mouth each day versus how little exercise I was doing that everything suddenly became clear."

One day, after I had given a lecture on weight loss in Brussels, a man raised his hand and asked me, "Why is it so difficult to change my eating habits? I'm really trying hard!"

I smiled. "Because you don't know them," I replied.

"What do you mean? I know what I eat!"

I smiled again. "What you eat doesn't define your eating habits, or only partially. It is how you eat and why you eat that way."

The man looked cross. "I know what I eat and why. I'm a grown-up!"

I spoke to him afterward and invited him to fill in the Food and Emotions Diary for a week. When we saw each other the following week he admitted that he had found it revelatory and had been having so many misconceptions about his eating habits.

As I have discussed, the truth is we tend to lie to ourselves in order to sabotage what we are doing and avoid making the changes we need to. We'd like to eat more healthily but, until we face the reality about our emotional needs for food, we're unable to do anything about it.

The aim of the diary is to give us a clear view of ourselves. You can see what I mean if you closely scrutinize Sophie's and Robert's diaries from Week One and then Week Four, after a month of filling them in daily. Many of you might be tempted just to look at what they ate and drank. This is natural – to compare ourselves to others and see if we eat in a similar way.

Knowing this, now take a look at the bigger picture – the one you don't yet have – about your own eating habits. Try to do this without comparing their patterns to yours, even though I know that is hard. Can you see the changes in the diaries between Week One and Week Four? We tend to see things in black or white, as good or bad, but being like that makes us very judgmental, preventing us from appreciating that long-term changes have to be made, step by step, in order for a new way of life to become truly sustainable.

Only when we get used to the changes can we cognitively accept each one and move on to the next. You may think that the difference between the diaries before and after is not that dramatic, and you'd be right. And the reason they are not so very different is because this means it can be sustainable for Sophie and Robert to move safely toward a way of eating and drinking which changes their weight (and their lives).

So ask yourself the following, writing down your answers:

▓ What are the changes I need to make in order to eat more healthily?

▓ Which ones should I start with?

▓ Should the bigger issues be the ones I address first?

▓ How will I begin?

Don't try to change anything about your eating habits during the first week. That way you can have a realistic view of when and where you eat, how much you eat, and why you eat the way you do. Of course, if by writing things down you realize that you don't want to finish your plate, or by being more mindful you choose a different kind of food, then go with the flow. It's not unusual for my clients to make some changes in the first week even if I'm not expecting any. In doing so, they are making choices that are no longer influenced by their emotions or their beliefs, and that's an encouraging start.

Some people will even put on weight during the first week, as they know that things are going to change and they unconsciously want to have a "final fling" and hold on to their habits for a bit longer, because what is familiar often feels much safer.

Each time you find an excuse not to fill in your diary is potentially another sabotage attempt. You may be tempted to justify this by telling yourself "I forgot," or "I didn't have enough time." I've even heard clients tell me, "I didn't write it down but I did it in my head."

If you do this too, then you will only be fooling yourself, which you've probably done many times in the past. If that happens, don't feel bad about it, just get back to the diary at the next meal or the following day. That way you will slowly build up a connection with your senses and your emotions that will boost your confidence. So remember, it's not a straight path, but as long as you stay on it you'll get there. I encourage you not to share anything you write, as it's very private. Friends, relatives and colleagues will all come up with advice they've read, or start to share their own struggles with food. But at this point you don't need their input. Instead, focus on yourself – a few minutes a day, a few times a day, not more.

Once you start filling in your own diary, it should become entirely natural and convenient to do. Many of my clients complete their diary on their phone or tablet and others on their laptop. Some buy lovely notebooks and write it all up by hand. You can also print out the sheets if you feel it's easier for you to use the grid in the examples. It doesn't matter, as long as you don't forget any information – and, most of all, if you do it when you're about to eat and while eating: in the moment, not retrospectively. Be mindful of your pace as well, as I mentioned before. It makes a real difference.

"You read about the modern hunger for 'life coaching' and think it's all a load of mumbo-jumbo for idiots, but when you start to be your own life coach it all makes sense. You don't have to go anywhere or see anyone. You can figure out all this stuff in your own head, in your own time and at your own pace. Genius."

In completing your Food and Emotions Diary, you will start to examine your eating habits more critically. You need to do this in a gentle way; it shouldn't be another occasion to judge yourself.

At this stage you start being your own coach, so you have to understand what you're doing wrong and come up with solutions.

Patterns will start to emerge in your own life that will allow you to appreciate that you eat in different ways with different companions or in a particular place. Most people find this immediately helpful. Best of all, they find out if they're really hungry or not at every meal.

Interestingly, just by doing this simple exercise every day you will find that you are more mindful about everything, usually with enormous benefits to your life generally. I hear that from my clients every day.

You may write, for example, that you were cross with your partner on Monday morning for not doing something you asked, which put you in a bad mood before you even had your breakfast. During the course of the week you might realize that this is a common annoyance for you, and one that often leads to you overeat. This realization can allow you to see the bigger picture of what may be affecting your happiness in your relationship and help you address the issue so that it doesn't remain as a bad habit.

Or you might see that at approximately 4pm every day you reach for a snack or something sweet to have with your tea because you are tired and your blood sugar is low. If this is a regular occurrence, then you will be eating hundreds of unwanted calories every day on top of your regular meals, which will quickly pile on the pounds. This realization may help you understand that you need to go to bed earlier at night or try to improve the quality of your sleep, so that you are less exhausted by the middle of the afternoon. Or you might take some fruit or a healthy snack to work with you to eat instead of a piece of cake or a sugary doughnut.

Before you start filling in the diary regularly, I'm pretty sure you'll be convinced you know everything about your eating habits – just like the man who challenged me in Brussels – so allow yourself to be surprised.

I am not a mindfulness guru by any means, but I do know that to stop and take a breath, or to review our week using tools like this diary, can give us a fresh perspective on our habits and help us transform them. Experts sometimes refer to this process as "looking down from the balcony", allowing us to rise above our everyday routines and examine them critically with an overview so that we can better assess how to improve them.

Many of my clients use this diary and get to the "balcony" and tell me that it has helped them so much that they are going to change their way of eating and make some important decisions about bringing mindfulness into their lives. "That's great!" I tell them, genuinely happy for them. "So, what are you going to do?"

Their faces often fall. "Well, I'm going to buy healthy food for the fridge instead of having takeaways all the time," they might say vaguely. Or, "I'm going to make a salad to take to work every day."

"Fantastic. What are you going to buy and when? When will you prepare it? The night before, or when you get up in the morning?"

It isn't good enough for us to simply decide that we will make these life-changing choices; we have to be realistic about what they involve and how we will manage them. There are some basic practicalities to consider. Fresh food has to be organized. Will it match our budget, for example? People often think that buying fresh and cooking fresh will be more expensive and take more time, but popular chefs have dispelled that myth. Buying your own food is often far less expensive than constantly paying for takeaways or processed meals. Cooking at home can take minutes and the very process of buying, washing, chopping and preparing your food is a kind of mindfulness itself, and a great way to fully appreciate how much you really want to consume and how hungry you are.

Changing habits isn't easy, but once a habit has been changed then it becomes a way of life that is easy to adhere to. You will have a new appreciation for what you are putting in your body and may even develop a taste for more sophisticated foods that are flavoursome and healthy at the same time.

The Food and Emotions Diary is a vital tool in understanding your own eating habits and patterns. It will help enhance your self-awareness and lead you to a more mindful way of life. The choice is yours.

TO RECAP

● Be gentle with yourself, not judgmental.

● See the patterns that emerge and address them.

● Don't try to change everything at once. Do it step by step.

● Be aware of how your position, environment, company and emotions affect your eating habits.

● Decide to make changes and then think about how to achieve them.

● Enjoy the difference being mindful, positive and intuitive makes to your life.

6

CONTROL YOUR LIFE – DON'T LET IT CONTROL YOU

"It was only when I was diagnosed with Type 2 diabetes that I finally realized I had to find the time to take better care of myself. I was angry and upset that I had let myself get that far. What could possibly be more important than my health?"

Our way of life plays a huge role when it comes to our food and drink issues. Most of us complain about being too tired or too busy, both of which prevent us from being able to accomplish everything we'd like.

People often dream of having a very different kind of life, hence the popularity of books, Instagram feeds and television programmes about the "slow food" movement, moving abroad or "escaping" to the country. So many people are unhappy in their careers and their relationships, or feel trapped by financial or other limitations. They spend so much of their lives commuting and/or under pressure at home and at work that managing their stress levels is their biggest challenge of the day.

Eating and drinking habits can be profoundly affected by this hurried and harried way of life. Frenetic schedules often lead to frenetic food intake, and to a way of eating that is far from mindful in nature. Cooking from scratch doesn't seem feasible and we may rely instead on processed food, constant snacking, takeaways or meals out. Some days we might binge and have a blowout meal, and on others we may not eat properly at all.

Yet, even though we know and accept the truth of how unhealthy our routine is, many people still believe that it is impossible to eat sensibly with the way of life they have.

There are five key questions to ask:

■ Where does this feeling that you are constantly running out of time come from?

- Who sets your schedule?

- What are you really spending your time on?

- What are the long-term health consequences if you continue on this path?

- How can you manage this differently?

My clients often arrive at their sessions with me a little late, breathless and stressed. They are apologetic and full of angst. "I've had a crazy day! The only thing that's kept me going is two bars of chocolate and an energy drink." Or, "I don't know where the time went today. I started early to get everything done but then the day conspired against me."

"Did it really?" I ask. "How so?" When I question them further I can usually help them to see that they are not nearly as busy as they think they are. They just *feel* that way because of the bad habits they have developed over the years.

So many people tell me that the first thing they do in the morning is reach for their phones. They don't allow themselves to wake gradually, get up, shower, have a coffee and think about their day. There is no pondering. No contemplation. No planning. From the moment their eyes are open they start trawling through their emails – work and personal – scrolling through social media to see what everyone else is doing (often making comparisons with their own life with some envy or resentment), and this continues throughout their hastily consumed breakfast and their morning commute to work, or while they are getting the children off to school.

By the time they officially start their working day – whatever that work may be – they have already been "working" for maybe three hours. And the whole day still stretches ahead of them – a day in which they are surrounded by friends, relatives and colleagues who mostly feel the same way and compete with each other over how busy and stressed they are.

Even during their so-called lunch or tea breaks, they remain connected to their devices and – therefore – to work, or to whichever demands people make of them. The expectation to respond immediately presses heavily on them, interrupting whatever they're doing as soon as they are alerted to a new message. This, in turn, impinges on the time they have to think about how hungry they are and what they might like to eat.

And when the day's work is finished, many of them choose to go out for drinks with their colleagues before going home. This may be their only recreational activity of the day, but it can also extend and expand stress even further, adding to the business of it all as they remain in work mode, discussing and complaining about their day. Drinking alcohol makes them hungry for unhealthy foods such as salty snacks and, on their commute home, they are still "hooked up" to the world, often buying more drinks and snacks almost on autopilot to eat on their journey.

By the time they reach home, they feel exhausted and stressed. They have been on the go since early that morning, and are usually too tired to cook a good meal or focus on how much they might consume. After grabbing something to eat they consider "quick and easy" such as a ready meal or a takeaway, they often remain connected to their colleagues, friends and family – while having the television on constantly in the background – until they go to bed, when their minds are racing so much that they cannot easily get to sleep.

The following day, the pattern simply repeats.

I see so many people on the brink of burning out, and have advised several to seek immediate medical help and get themselves signed off from work. They didn't seem to recognize the warning signs and needed me to get them to take the next step. Coming to me probably was their next step, but – once again – it goes back to the ego states of Child, Parent and Adult (see page 39). In a situation like that, the client wanted me to be the Parent and tell them what to do, which meant that he or she could be the Child. Had they summoned their inner Adult, they would have been able to take that decision for themselves, but being the Child allowed them to remain helpless and absolved of any responsibility for their own way of life and actions.

When my clients are late to my sessions, they often tell me, "I'm so sorry. I'm sure you're as busy as I am." I look at them and smile before saying, "No, not really," which always takes them aback.

"Yes," I add, "I have many clients and could have even more, but the difference is that I make sure I have time to myself each day. I stay off my devices and avoid the television; I allow myself the time and space to wake up properly and breathe and think about my day. I go for a walk or read a book or listen to some music. I plan my meals, shop, prepare and cook them. These are the times that I keep just for me, not for anyone else, and they are what give me the feeling of calmness that allows me to face the rest of my day."

When they express their envy at the way I manage my way of life, telling me, "Gee, you're so lucky you can live that way!" I confess that things weren't always like that for me, until I made the decision to master my own life.

Gently, I tell them, "You could live like this too. You just have to make the decision to change." For many this comes as a complete revelation.

"From the moment I wake to the moment I go to sleep I am ruled by lists. They're everywhere – by my bed, on my phone, pinned to the fridge, at my desk. I never complete any of them and when I eventually go to bed I fall asleep but wake at 4am with more 'To-Dos' in my head, so I turn on the light and write another list."

Just as we did with the Food and Emotions Diary (see Chapter 5), I want you to write down how many minutes or hours you spend on every activity during an average day. This will enable you to "go to the balcony" again (see page 154–5) and look at the bigger picture. You'll be surprised by how much time you spend doing some of the activities you do without thinking almost every day.

Here is the example of someone I'll call Steve:

07:00	Woke with alarm clock/radio. Blaring music. Reached for phone. Surfed and answered emails – 15 minutes.
07:15	Turned on TV to watch breakfast telly – 5 minutes. Checked phone throughout.
07:20	Showered and shaved – 8 minutes. Checked emails and social media again – 5 minutes. Watched TV while changing for work – 10 minutes.
07:45	Ate a bowl of cereal and a piece of toast and marmalade with coffee – 10 minutes.
07:55	Walked to the station and caught the 08.15 train. Checked emails and social media along the way – 20 minutes.

08:15	Standing room only on train so plugged in earphones and watched an episode of my favourite show – 30 minutes.
08:45	Walked to office – 15 minutes. Picked up a sausage roll and a latte – 5 minutes.
09:05	Sat at my desk, ate sausage roll and drank coffee. Chatted to colleague – 5 minutes. Went to the bathroom – 5 minutes.
09:15	Started work. Busy day. Took a lot of calls. Felt stressed – 135 minutes.
11:30	Took a break. Made myself a cup of tea and ate two cookies. Checked emails and social media – 15 minutes.
11:45	Worked on. Still busy – 90 minutes.
13:15	Decided to eat a sandwich at my desk for lunch as it was raining. Bought it from the canteen with a can of cola – 15 minutes.
13:30	Spent the rest of my lunch break online, buying some new shoes and stuff for my car – 30 minutes.
14:00	Work relentless. Lots of calls and paperwork. Tired and under pressure – 90 minutes.
15:30	Cup of tea in the canteen and a piece of flapjack. Surfed the internet – 15 minutes.

15:45	Less than two hours to go. Not as busy with work, so read the newspaper in the bathroom and listened to some music with my earphones for 10 minutes – 105 minutes in all.
17:30	Off to the bar with some of my friends, drank two beers and ate a bag of peanuts – 60 minutes.
18:30	Train home, got a seat, played a game online. Made the journey seem faster – 30 minutes.
19:00	Poured myself a glass of wine when I got in and reheated the leftovers of last night's curry – 10 minutes.
19:10	Turned TV on and slumped on sofa watching it as well as making calls and answering emails – 110 minutes.
21:00	Binge-watched two episodes of a series I've been following. Ate the last of the leftovers and had more wine – 120 minutes.
23:00	Went to bed, checked emails and watched funny YouTube videos on my iPad before setting the alarm – 20 minutes.
03:15	Wide awake, heart racing. Drank some water and trawled through Instagram until bored and sleepy – 20 minutes.

In this example, Steve spends approximately 420 minutes (seven hours) doing what he would call work, which amounts to six hours. By contrast, he spends 445 minutes or seven and a half hours online, watching television or playing a computer game. The time he devotes to eating and drinking is approximately two hours, and even then he is doing something else. The rest of his time is taken up with showering and commuting.

Because he has not set himself clear barriers between work and play, Steve has led himself to believe that he works really hard and is always busy. In fact, that isn't the case. His feelings come more from the pressure and tension he places himself under by allowing his work to permeate the whole of his day, from the moment he wakes to the moment he goes to sleep. If we can become better connected to ourselves and respectful of our own feelings all day long, then the whole day becomes "me time".

If Steve were to halve his time online or watching television, for example, that would free up more than three hours every day in which he could get outside and enjoy nature, play sport, join a club, take up a hobby or socialize. Better still, he could shop, prepare and cook food that would be better for his overall wellbeing. Plus, he would probably sleep better and be less tired all day.

People talk about their dreams of leading a better, bigger life than the one they have in a way that makes it sound like it's completely unattainable – or certainly far too difficult to fit into their schedule – when it would actually have huge benefits. Finding "me time" to do something that doesn't revolve around eating and drinking is the best thing you can do for your general wellbeing, and for weight loss.

Why can't you learn how to play the guitar, or go to a language class, or join a book club? What is stopping you? Could it be you?

Now here is the diary of someone I will call Helen:

05:00	Woke to the sound of the baby crying. Tended to him and took him downstairs for his bottle. Made a cup of tea and ate three cookies while listening to the radio – 90 minutes.
06:30	My partner woke up and took over caring for the baby so I could have a shower and get dressed – 20 minutes. Our four-year-old daughter got up and climbed into our bed. I turned on the TV so she could watch breakfast telly while I checked my phone for emails and social media – 10 minutes.
07:00	Put the baby in his cot and made breakfast of porridge and toast for my partner and daughter – 30 minutes. Checked emails and social media again – 5 minutes. Watched kids' TV while washing up – 10 minutes. My partner left for work.
07:45	Ate a piece of cold buttered toast, the leftover bowl of cereal, and finished up the porridge in the pan – 30 minutes.
08:15	Dressed my daughter and put the baby in his buggy and the dog on a lead. Left the house and walked my daughter to school – 25 minutes. Dropped her at school and chatted to some of the other mums before walking to the park to exercise the dog – and me – 20 minutes.

09:00 No other mums I knew were in the park so headed home via a café where I treated myself to a large cappuccino and a Danish pastry as I felt I deserved it. Took a photo of it for Instagram and surfed the internet on their free WiFi – 60 minutes.

10:00 Walked home, baby grizzly – 25 minutes. Fed him and put him down. Put a wash on. Sat down and tried to read the newspaper but got involved in an online chat about a friend's affair – 20 minutes. Checked social media – 10 minutes.

10:55 Went to my office and started sifting through the mail. Made a couple of calls and chatted to friends – 30 minutes.

11:25 Picked up a new project I had intended to start this week but felt too tired and overwhelmed. Hungry, I made myself a cheese sandwich – 20 minutes.

11:45 Lay on the sofa for a quick nap. Went out like a light and woke suddenly to hear the baby crying – 15 minutes. Brought him down and gave him a bottle, made myself a cup of tea and ate two chocolate cookies. Checked emails and social media – 15 minutes.

12:15 Decided to prepare and cook up some vegetables to mash for the baby, which took longer than I thought as I was watching an old movie – 75 minutes.

13:30 With the baby happy playing in his cot I took the baby alarm and went upstairs to make the beds and clean the bathroom – 40 minutes.

14:10	Hungry again so ate a banana and yoghurt. Drank it with a diet cola while watching daytime TV – 20 minutes.
14:30	Put the baby in the buggy, grabbed the dog and walked to my daughter's school to collect her – 30 minutes.
15:00	Chatted to the other mothers and kids – 15 minutes. Accepted an invitation to join them at a local café with a garden. Wasn't hungry but ate a ham and brie baguette – 60 minutes.
16:15	Walked home – 25 minutes. Made my daughter some tea and fed the baby – 30 minutes. While they were eating and playing I went online and bought a bunch of stuff and ordered some groceries to be delivered– 30 minutes. Then I got involved in an online chat with other parents about exhaustion – 30 minutes.
18:10	Bathed the baby (with the help of my daughter) and she had a bath and changed into her pyjamas. Put the baby down and my daughter to bed – 50 minutes.
19:00	A bit of "me time" before my partner comes home. He has promised to bring pizzas, so no cooking for me. Put some music on, opened some wine and spent time trawling through social media and trying not to be jealous of other people's lives. Hungry so ate a bag of crisps – 60 minutes.

20:00	Partner home with two giant pizzas. We finished the wine and ate the lot – 30 minutes. He immediately took to the sofa and his iPad to finish up some work stuff, and I felt resentful so I opened a second bottle of wine, poured myself a glass and had a hot bath – 30 minutes.
21:00	Partner asleep on sofa. I was too tired to stay up so went to bed. Sad.

In this example, Helen is genuinely busy with childcare in her 16-hour day but during that period she actually has approximately 10 hours to do what she likes. She uses that time to walk in the park, do some shopping, surf the internet, take a nap and have a hot bath. She is pretty good at balancing her "me time" but tends to eat on reflex because she feels she "deserves" it, or because it's convenient and she is tired.

Her food intake is very unhealthy – leftovers, pastries, baguettes, pizzas – all very heavy on the carbohydrates. Yet she spent quite a lot of time preparing healthy vegetables for her baby, not thinking to double them up and keep some back for herself and her partner. She also lost a lot of time on negative online chats or comparing her life to other people's which could have been spent instead doing something more beneficial for her own wellbeing and sense of worth.

Look at your own patterns and see where you can make time savings. If, for example, you discover that you are spending far more time than you thought playing computer games, or watching mindless television, then decide how to spend those precious minutes focusing on things that are more beneficial for you such as gardening, socializing or having good times with your family. And when it comes to preparing food, enjoy the extra time you now have to think about what you will eat, how hungry you are, and to notice when you are full.

> "Every day I tell myself that tomorrow I will be better, eat better, do better and find myself some time just for me. Then the next day comes and, guess what, I just repeat the same bad habits over and over, as if I am on some kind of self-destructive loop. Well, I need to cut the loop."

Feeling that we never have enough time gives us the perfect excuse to avoid making changes in our lives. It is also a way of perpetuating the myth that life always has to be a struggle – a daily fight – when this isn't true at all.

Of course, for some people it is: those with physical or psychological disabilities, those who are struggling financially, and others who have problems with relationships or a troubled family history. For most of us, though, there are a myriad of choices about how we live, where we live, who we associate with and what we do.

We may feel guilty about earning more than others, or the homes that we live in compared to the majority of the world. We may want to let everyone know how hard we have worked to earn these perks of our labours, or we may be harbouring emotions from our childhood that compel us to complain and play the victim all the time.

For that is the benefit of constantly moaning about how busy you are – you become the "victim" of the system, your workplace, your family, your boss or your life (see opposite). It's not your fault you're so tired or stressed. It's everyone else. You feel both helpless and hopeless. In Steve's case, the benefits of being this way are that he has an excuse not to see people or do things he doesn't want to, and being busy has become some kind of validation for his life – as it has for most of the people around him. He worries that, if he was to be chilled and relaxed while they constantly complained, then he might not be "one of them" anymore and could even be regarded as lazy. In truth, they would admire him and he might even inspire them to make similar changes in their own lives.

Being the victim also absolves him from being put upon further by anyone. "We can't ask Steve to coach the five-a-side team. He's knackered enough already from his job." It puts the onus on others to give you sympathy, or to be impressed by how well you function despite all your trials and tribulations. "Helen's amazing. She cooks all her children's food from organic vegetables rather than buying it in jars like the rest of us." How do people even know that? Because Helen is sure to tell them that she does, and how long it takes.

Victim Complex

Victim Complex or Victim Mentality is defined as an acquired personality trait in which the individual frequently or constantly adopts a "poor me" attitude to life, seeing themselves as the victims of everybody else's actions. This trait often stems from childhood experiences where they felt helpless and under the control of someone in authority, be it a sibling, a parent or another adult. In such cases, the victim convinces himself or herself that they are blameless for events that happen to them and deserve sympathy and understanding from those around them.

Have a look at the following list and ask yourself, which benefits do you gain from always feeling tired and stressed and overworked – and then telling everyone about it?

- sympathy

- compassion

- impressing people

- gain in stature

- leeway

Whenever we feel afraid to make changes in our life, we can sabotage ourselves in a thousand or more ways. Being too tired or too busy is probably the excuse I hear most often, but there are so many others. The human brain is extremely inventive when it comes to getting us off the hook:

- "I want to have a healthier way of life but my family would walk out if I started serving them salad every night."

- "I can't afford any more cookery books and, anyway, I have nowhere to put them."

- "Changing my whole way of life is just too difficult for me right now. Maybe next year when things are calmer."

- "I'm known as Freddie Fries. It's become a joke and all my friends call me that. If I stop eating fries at every meal, what will they call me then?"

Even something as apparently unrelated as the weather plays a surprisingly important role in the amount and timing of our intake. So often I hear clients tell me, "Oh, it was so cold and wet that evening that I drank a couple of Irish coffees to warm me up." I nod and smile and say, "Wouldn't a cup of tea or coffee have worked just as well?"

Then when the sun comes out, they say, "It was so hot and sunny, it was perfect weather to drink a bottle of rosé." I smile and quietly tell them, "Let's hope it rains tomorrow then."

When I gently tease them like this, they're often shocked to realize how nonsensical their justification sounds. We can all make up wild excuses for our lapses over food and drink, and sometimes it's only when we express them in writing or speech that we realize how shallow they are.

Holidays often feel like the most difficult times for people who are trying to be mindful of what they eat. The feeling of entitlement to have a good time is the natural response to the sense of being overworked and overstressed all the time. Whenever we're away from our work or everyday environment, it is easy to get into the mentality of, "We can drink and eat all we want. We're on holiday!"

These are the kinds of things my clients tell me:

- "We had such a great vacation but I put on 6 kilos (1 stone). We ate a huge breakfast at the hotel buffet each morning, then went to the taverna for lunch every day, and still had dinner out each evening. Plus we drank most of the day and really got into the cocktails at night. I told my husband, the diet starts tomorrow."

- "I hardly ever get time to see my family so it was great to treat them to meals out every day and eat ice creams by the pool and to drink a bit more without being worried about work or driving home. I deserve that."

▓ "My partner and I are like ships passing in the night these days and it wasn't easy to spend every day together. We don't have much in common anymore so eating was the only time we shared anything enjoyable together."

▓ "Although I was looking forward to my holiday, I didn't enjoy it so much. The lads I went with just wanted to get drunk every night, and I had to join in. I woke every morning with a horrible hangover and felt sick because I'd eaten and drunk so much the previous night."

▓ "I gained 5 kilos (10 pounds) because I couldn't help but pick at the kids' food as well as my own. Unlike at home, they almost always ordered something fried and those chips were just too much of a temptation."

With these kinds of responses there's a sense of resignation: people feel they are helpless and have no choice but to overindulge on holiday. But it doesn't have to be that way. One client of mine had a big family event coming up for which she wanted to lose weight, although she had already lost a good deal.

"I'm going to get a new dress and hat and I want to look great for the photographs," she told me excitedly. Then her face fell. "The trouble is, I'm going to France for two weeks just before, which will be terrible for my diet!"

"Will it?" I asked. "Why?"

"Oh, you know, all that lovely French wine and bread and cheese. It'll be so tempting."

"And there's no reason why you can't have some of it, *if* and *when* you are hungry, stopping when you are full," I reminded her.

Her face lit up as she suddenly realized that she could continue with her new way of life away in France as easily as she could when she was at home.

People often don't seem to realize that being on holiday is actually one of the best places to lose weight. There is usually good-quality food on offer with several healthy options on the menu. If you are in a hotel, you won't even have to cook it, so there'll be no temptation to eat while you cook. If you are somewhere warm and sunny, then you can swim or cycle, go for a hike, ride a horse and generally be more active than you might be at home.

All that extra cardiovascular activity coupled with a greater choice of food and wine means that you can build up your appetite then relax, enjoy your break and eat mindfully without any sense of guilt.

> **"I never thought I'd lose weight on holiday, but we walked 3 miles in the hills each morning and then I chose fruit and protein for breakfast. I was in the pool all morning and then ate a delicious salad for lunch. In the afternoons we read and dozed before walking to the harbour for supper instead of taking a cab. I couldn't believe I'd lost 3 kilos (half a stone)!"**

Sleep deprivation is another big issue for weight loss because if we don't sleep enough we are far more tempted to eat more sugar and carbohydrates. Almost all of my clients complain of fatigue. They either can't sleep, or don't sleep well, and a surprisingly high number frequently take both medication for insomnia and the "smart drugs" popular with students for boosting energy and concentration.

Many tell me about waking up in the middle of the night with their hearts racing and their minds in a state of high anxiety. Every worry they have ever had seems to crowd their thoughts and they often feel the need to get up and make themselves something to eat or drink to "calm" them down, often taking to the internet to distract them from their unhappy thoughts. It is such a common problem. Just take a look at social media and you will be amazed by how many pages or hashtags there are that begin with: *3amthoughts*.

I am not a sleep expert but I have experienced many sleepless nights in my life, like everyone else. I can completely relate to the patterns that I see emerging from the stories my clients tell me. Like many of them, I wear a device on my wrist that tells me how many hours I slept and how much of that I was in the deepest, REM (rapid eye movement) sleep. Unlike many of them, though, I try not to obsess about it.

"I had only 30 minutes' deep sleep last night. No wonder I'm tired," clients tell me, or "Last night was my sixth disturbed night in a row so I feel very grumpy."

For those who have a chronic problem, I suggest they speak to their doctor or even go to a specialist clinic for overnight monitoring to see what is affecting their sleep patterns. Some people have the opposite problem. They sleep too much. Fatigue is a common symptom of depression, a way of putting our emotions to sleep, and it may be that the person is depressed or in need of some counselling to help them through a difficult period.

Most people don't need to visit a specialist clinic or see a therapist though. They just need to make themselves aware of their own actions and habits in order to make some simple changes that will have lasting effects.

Just as with the previous diaries, it is helpful to write down your sleep patterns over an average week, taking special note of your activities in the hours before you go to bed. Look at the example below of three days in the life of someone I will call Joe:

JOE'S SLEEP DIARY

Monday:

19:30	Home from work, ate supper (pasta).
20:00	Took a shower, changed and sent a few emails.
20:45	Watched a movie with my partner. Ate popcorn and chocolate.
23:00	Partner went to bed. Although tired, I stayed up to surf the internet.
23:55	Indigestion so made a hot drink and watched TV.
01:30	Went to bed, fell straight asleep.
03:45	Wide awake. Worries about work and money.
04:10	Got up and made hot chocolate and ate 3 cookies.
04:50	Back to bed, finally drifted off.
06:30	Alarm woke me. Felt exhausted.

Tuesday:

19:00	Met partner in town for supper with friends. Ate and drank too much.
22:00	Went to a bar afterward for nightcap. Ended up being two.
23:00	Home but buzzing. Partner went to bed. I played computer game.
Midnight:	Went to bed but couldn't sleep. Put bedroom TV on. Mind racing.
01:15	Finally went to sleep.
04:00	Wide awake again, needed the toilet. Felt hungover.
04:45	Back to sleep.
06:30	Alarm. Exhausted.

Wednesday:

19:30	Home from work with takeaway Chinese.
20:00	Showered, changed, surfed internet and watched a horrible programme on Syria.
21:00	Watched three episodes of *Game of Thrones*. We both fell asleep.

Midnight:	Went to bed. Immediately asleep.
05:00	Woken by nightmare after *Game of Thrones*. Woke partner. Watched some TV.
05:45	Back to sleep.
06:30	Alarm. Exhausted.

Looking at Joe's diary, it is clear that he is staying up too late after a day's work, and overindulging in his use of technology at night. Sleep experts advise against having any televisions, telephones or computers in the bedroom and to avoid them for an hour before bedtime. He should also be mindful of the influence of the media on our anxiety and how it can give us a negative view of the world.

Nor is Joe mindful enough of the kinds of things that he is eating and drinking too close to bedtime. Alcohol and chocolate, takeaways and too many carbohydrates will only raise his blood pressure and increase his heart rate. Doing some exercise after his meal, such as going for a walk or playing sport, would also help him digest his food and tire him physically. Having a hot bath or spending some time in quiet contemplation – meditating, reading, listening to soothing music – can also help in quietening the mind in preparation for sleeping.

Some people consciously or subconsciously delay the moment they turn the lights off because they feel like they want to squeeze more out of their day; almost as if they want a second day. Others find it difficult to go to bed because they fear it will increase their sensation of loneliness. Many delay bedtime because they're afraid that they won't fall asleep until they're completely exhausted. In every case it's worth addressing these issues of loneliness and anxiety, otherwise things will only get worse.

By making ourselves aware of these patterns we can make simple changes, such as getting an early night two or three times a week and being careful what we do, what we eat and what we drink. Awareness of environmental effects combined with healthy eating habits is vital to achieving a good night's sleep.

> **"I feel as if I have been suffering from exhaustion for the last ten years. I can hardly remember the last time I had a good night's sleep. I wake up more tired than when I went to bed and spend much of the day yawning. I know I am older than I was when I had unlimited energy but I'd love not to feel like this all the time."**

We are all bombarded by media and advertising campaigns telling us how to lead our lives and what kinds of things we should or shouldn't be doing. A few of them are helpful and offer good advice. Most aren't. Some are more obvious than others, and the use of subliminal advertising to influence our way of life is something we should all be wary of.

Whenever we enter a supermarket, for example, some of the first items we are usually offered are sandwiches or chocolates, often on a "buy one get one free" promotion or priced at a discount. Thus begins the temptation, especially if the reason we are there in the first place is to buy food for our next meal because we're hungry.

This kind of commercialization continues throughout the store, right to the checkout in order to tempt us again. Chocolates and other confectionery are on display at almost every cashier's station, to tempt us still further. The same is true for petrol or filling stations, bookstores, even toy stores. Temptation is everywhere and can be difficult to resist, even more so for the children who sometimes accompany us when we go shopping. We are not going to change the way these stores do their merchandising, but it is good to be aware of their strategies in order to make more reasonable choices. Keep in mind that the omnipresence of these items does not make them more legitimate.

The way we buy and the way we eat is a sad indictment of our consumerist society. People are obsessed with acquisition – they need to buy more, have more, eat more, drink more (the more unusual and exotic the better). They often do this because they are constantly comparing themselves to those who have all the things they want but can't really afford. Someone clever called it "affluenza", a word that implies that our increasing affluence has become an epidemic or disease. In a way, it has. We don't need all that stuff, all those clothes or all that food. It's hardly surprising that there is so much interest at the moment in the "decluttering" movement, trying to get people back to a simple, less voracious way of life.

Nor do we have to be swayed by advertising or media campaigns that can hoodwink us into buying less than healthy foods. I am not a dietician, but in my opinion the sugar lobbies and the food industry have a lot to answer for. We only have to read the small print on the labels of so-called "diet foods" to discover that they may be low in fat, but are laden with sugars, or vice versa. Blaming the food industry, though, isn't the solution. We each have to take responsibility for our food choices. We want things to be easy to prepare (or already prepared) and we're not always ready to change our habits. We then pay the price for this easier way of life, which isn't that easy anymore when our weight goes up.

I know it is easier and more convenient to do all your shopping in the same supermarket, but I strongly encourage you to visit your local market when you can, or buy products direct from the farm and delivered to your door. In this way we can buy quality products at reasonable prices from people who will often be happy to tell us about their produce. Aside from being more environmentally friendly, it allows us to be much more in touch with what we are going eat and with those who are providing it. We don't have to always buy a bag of salad or a shrink-wrapped piece of meat, which completely disconnects us from what we are going to eat. We can buy fresh fruits and vegetables whose provenance we know, or meat from a butcher who can talk to us with enthusiasm about its source. If you have a garden or even a window box, you can grow your own.

We have dehumanized food, like so many other things, and this distance between it and us plays an important role in the way we feed ourselves. In order to reverse that dehumanization, we can take up cooking in a way that is fun and interesting and gives us back control of what we are putting into our mouths. It doesn't have to be anything too complicated. There is a plethora of cookbooks and television programmes specializing in quick and simple recipes these days.

It is not uncommon that, full of good intentions, we buy a new cookbook only to make as little use of it as we do of our gym membership (which was my case, to be honest). This can discourage us even more. If you have lost self-confidence and forgotten how to cook, then why not take some cookery classes to refamiliarize yourself with your culinary skills. It can also be another opportunity to meet new people who have also decided to be more proactive and responsible. This will put you in a more positive state of mind and make you more aware of what you eat.

Some may worry about the financial cost of these initiatives, but this will ultimately prove more economical than you may have imagined. I have enthusiastic clients who have gone a step farther and even taken the initiative to teach cookery classes in local schools to familiarize children with healthier eating patterns. When you get back to cooking, involve your children. It will be an experience they won't forget and one that can be of great help to them in their adult life.

"I can't believe the junk I used to give my family. Bread laden with fat and sugar, processed foods rich in additives and salt. Now I look forward to shopping, cooking and eating the food I buy, happy in the knowledge that it's chemical-free plus I am supporting local farmers. It's a win-win."

The overuse of vitamin and mineral food supplements makes me especially mad. A recent study found that an alarming number didn't even contain the ingredients they claimed to. Taking handfuls of those, as so many of my friends and clients do, leads in my opinion only to an expensive *pisse*! It's all about clever marketing.

Detoxing is another largely fraudulent process. If we have an indulgent few days of eating and drinking, then eating healthily for a few days afterward is all we need to do. We certainly don't need to deprive our body of food, which will lead only to low blood sugar, insatiable hunger and excessive binge eating.

In my opinion, all these fads are creating an epidemic of eating disorders, many of which I spend my working day dealing with. I witness so much pain and distress – and not only from adults. I see teenagers in conflict with parents who've sent them to me to address their weight issues, at a time when they should be having fun and not be full of angst about what size skinny jeans they can get into. Many of them fear they are facing a lifetime of dieting like their parents.

It's not clever and it's becoming a serious issue. I am at my most assertive about food when something endangers my clients and jeopardizes their relationships with happiness. This issue of indoctrination in society is definitely one that needs to be addressed.

In order to bring about any long-lasting change, the biggest change we have to make is to acknowledge that for the first time things can truly be different. We don't have to be trapped in a body that we don't like or even recognize. We have been locked in a system that we created and we are the only ones with the key to our own freedom.

TO RECAP

- A frenetic way of life almost always means frenetic eating. No matter how busy you are, you can make time to eat mindfully, so keep a time diary and allow yourself the pleasure and space to do so.

- Remind yourself who sets your schedule and don't ignore the long-term risks to your health of burning out.

- Set clear boundaries between work and play. Use your time diary to see where savings can be made.

- Be the Adult, not the Child. Accept responsibility for your life and make the decision to change bad habits.

- Don't play the victim all your life. Acknowledge the benefits to you of no longer doing so.

- Stop making excuses about holidays and the weather to justify overeating.

- Pay attention to your sleep patterns and address any issues that are disturbing them.

- Be aware of how advertising and the media can influence what foods you buy. Get back to shopping for fresh produce and enjoy its preparation.

CASE STUDY

Claire frequently arrived late for our first sessions. Breathlessly she would then offer various excuses - blaming public transport, her job, her boss, her colleagues and so on. In short, she gave me a list of all those who she felt had contributed to her delay without ever accepting any personal responsibility. Her shortness of breath proved to me that she had hurried and made me more feel more forgiving, although I wasn't there to judge her but to find solutions, adult to adult.

I could see that my passive response to her repeated lateness confused her because she expected anger or disappointment, responses she generally received from others for her lack of punctuality. The persona she had developed as a "victim" generally sparked a saviour or prosecutor reaction in others. She was either pitied or insulted. This classic mode of operation had been hers since she was very young and she had locked herself into that scenario, which only damaged the quality of her relationships with others. It was also boring and repetitive for her (and for them).

I was able to help her see the toxic effects this could have on her relationships and on her life in general. I invited her to experiment on a daily basis with being more responsible and more mature in her relationships, starting with her relationship with herself. No longer pretending to be a victim was like a revelation to her. Once she overcame her fear of the consequences that a change in her behaviour might bring, Claire was able to get out of this negative model and become fully responsible for her own actions. This change in her attitude allowed her to make real choices, far beyond those that concerned punctuality, food and drink. These are not always easy choices, but they are certainly choices that can allow you to live your life better and in full awareness.

7

WILL DRINKING LESS MAKE YOU BORED – AND BORING?

> "I get it about not eating unless I'm hungry, but I'm finding it really difficult not to drink so much. I know it's all extra calories, but I just can't give up that great feeling of relaxation that a few glasses of wine bring me at the end of the day."

Alcohol is omnipresent in our society, which often glamorizes it in various ways. Temptation is everywhere, offering us a sense of warm familiarity. It has come to feel completely normal to spend an evening drinking with friends, or on our own. We can always rely on alcohol to make things better, can't we?

Until it starts making things worse.

One of the first things a host asks when you walk into their home is, "What can I get you to drink?" It's the same with staff when you enter a bar or restaurant. Pubs and bars now have lists of gins as detailed as their food menus, while craft breweries and artisan distillers have captivated the hipster generation with their different flavoured alcohols. Adverts featuring "beautiful people" are plastered across our everyday environment, from television commercials to online ads or posters on the side of the bus. All of them use the best-looking models to persuade us that to eat this or drink that is cool and will make us one of them. Bombarded with so many pro-alcohol stimuli, is it a wonder that when we get home our bottles of cold beer or chilled white wine in the refrigerator seem especially enticing?

Because alcohol has become so pervasive in our culture, it is often what we turn to when we are feeling our most extreme emotions. Whenever we are happy we want to celebrate, and that almost always involves drinking with friends, family or colleagues. When we're sad we often drink to "drown our sorrows". When we are angry, we pour ourselves a "stiff drink" to calm down. Ditto when we are in shock or upset. For an alarmingly high number of people, it would feel rude or weird to abstain from drinking for an extended period of time. "What would people think if I gave up?" is something I hear commonly, such is the stigma surrounding alcoholism.

Drinking gives us the power of deflecting ourselves away from painful or uncomfortable experiences, as we feel it takes the edge off our day. For some of us, it can become like a relationship – a love affair even – a dependency that we cannot imagine living without. It comes with a plethora of enjoyable rituals that often involve camaraderie and some of our happiest moments. It can provide a safety net and give us courage. It can melt our anxieties. It can make us feel warm and friendly and sexy.

Getting tipsy can bring out the playful Child in us; the one you now know about from Transactional Analysis (see page 39). This Child gets excited by alcohol – even by the idea of it sometimes – and looks forward to how drink will enable it to express itself in a way it feels it might not be able to without the lubrication. Of course it is fun to be silly and stupid sometimes, to let our hair down and express ourselves. We don't need alcohol to do this, though. We can do it through play of other kinds – with our children, with our friends, with our lovers. I run an improvisation class and for two hours every week we act like giggly kids, creating crazy personas for ourselves and being quite ridiculous. And we do all that on tea or coffee, water or juice. No alcohol required.

The way alcohol takes a hold on us is a slow, insidious process. We are gradually drawn in and become committed to our relationship with it in a way that is different from almost any other. We know it's not good for us and we make promises that we'll stick to "Dry January" next year, or at least try not to drink for two or three nights a week, but then we are tempted by a friend or a situation or our dependency, and we crack and tell ourselves that we'll start again tomorrow.

For most of my life, I have enjoyed social drinking – with friends, family, lovers. I especially love fine wines and, as a restaurateur, used to take a lot of time and trouble to source the perfect wine to match the food. Nothing has changed. I still enjoy wine very much, just not as often, which – in a way – makes it all the more enjoyable. I usually stop drinking after two glasses and try to avoid situations where friends or colleagues meet in a pub or bar with the deliberate intention of drinking all night. To drink or not to drink is my choice. It is part of my decision to lead a healthier, happier life, to sleep better, to be fitter and not to overload my body with toxins.

This can be your choice too.

> **"When the doctor told me I had alarmingly high enzymes in my liver indicating early liver disease, I was so shocked. I am only 32 and never thought what I considered to be normal social drinking would have such an adverse effect."**

You would have to live on another planet not to know the impact that excessive alcohol consumption can have on our health, both physical and mental. The same media that often promotes alcohol repeatedly warns us of liver failure, diabetes and heart disease, to name but a few. The consequences of overconsumption can be dire and even deadly. And yet the alcohol market is thriving, despite some interesting initiatives from government and others to try to hold the public more accountable.

Aside from the damage excessive alcohol might be doing to their livers, for many of my clients it also has a massive influence on their weight problems. For some, in fact, this is the single most difficult obstacle in the way of achieving and maintaining a healthy size and shape. It is the last piece of territory they are prepared to concede.

They may be ready to change their eating habits, eat at a more appropriate pace, be attentive to their hunger, eat fewer pre-cooked products and reduce their consumption of sugars. But when I start talking about their alcohol consumption they tense up physically, and regard me suspiciously as the one who might be about to take away their greatest source of pleasure and sense of joy. Sometimes, it may be their only source of those things. And why is this? Because, according to them, drinking alcohol is "cool". They try to barter with me, saying, "But I'm so much more relaxed when I drink," or "We laugh more easily," or "I feel closer to others," or "It helps me disconnect from the worry of daily life."

Yes, just like all drugs do – but is it harmless?

Time and again a client will list in quite unnecessary detail what carbohydrates they've avoided the previous week, how they ate twice their "five a day" of fruit and vegetables, how many steps they walked, and the calories they burned. Then I ask them how many units of alcohol they drank and they shrug and say, "Three or four glasses of wine each night, but that's all part of the Mediterranean diet, right?" They don't fully appreciate (or they choose to ignore) the fact that each calorie gained from alcohol consumption also forms part of their daily calorific intake. It's simple but also complicated, because drinking has other damaging repercussions on your food intake, which we'll discuss in a minute.

One of my clients was extremely proud that she'd reduced her weekly alcohol intake from 70 to 40 units but still didn't appreciate that 40 units was too much. I reminded her that drinking adds unwanted calories on top of her food intake, which in turn adds weight, so if she carried on drinking to excess then, no matter how mindfully or intuitively she ate, the therapy would never work. If each glass of wine or beer we drink contributes inches to our waistlines then – no matter how mindful we are of what we're eating – the weight will never come off.

The answer rarely relies on giving up alcohol but instead on understanding our relationship with it and empowering ourselves to be more moderate. Needing a drink is something we can change. It is another kind of hunger – an emotional dependency. If we take alcohol away, then we need to think of other ways to unwind and cope with our stresses, fears and emotions. We need to pause and find out what's really going on.

The same gentle rules relating to our food intake also apply to drinking alcohol. Once we start to become more aware of what we are eating and drinking every day, we begin to realize that the third or fourth glass rarely tastes as good as the first or second, so why not stop there? Like so many of my clients, you will experience the joy of being back in control.

We also need to be aware of the many social triggers that play a huge part in our drinking habits. So here are some of them, plus some ways of handling how they make us feel:

- Drinking **to relax** – "God, I need a drink! I have a few every night to properly relax after my hectic day." Think of other ways to do that, such as having a hot bath, going for a run, playing some sort of game or sport, or listening to music.

- Drinking **to be part of the group** – "I can't imagine going to a bar and not drinking when all my friends are." If they are true friends, they should applaud your efforts to be healthier and may even be inspired by you.

- Drinking **to keep someone company** – "My friend won't feel like going out with me as she'll feel awkward drinking alone." If you take the initiative your friend may follow suit and also drink less.

Drinking **by way of reward** – "I feel like I deserve a few drinks for everything I've accomplished all day, it's my treat." Again, think of other ways to reward yourself – cook yourself a delicious meal, buy yourself some flowers, contact a friend or relative to share your sense of accomplishment.

Drinking so as **not to be seen as boring** – "My friends would tease me horribly if I said I wasn't drinking on a night out." Ignore them and they'll soon stop, or try teasing them back about their drinking.

Drinking **to relieve stress** – "It's tough out there. When I'm getting drunk I stop worrying about it." Take up yoga or meditation, go for a walk, or talk to a loved one about your worries. Go to the cinema, watch a comedy on television, or read a book. Find other means of relief, and remember that drinking will make you more stressed by ruining your sleep and damaging your self-confidence because of all the extra calories you drank.

Drinking **to appear smarter and funnier** – "I'm so much funnier when I'm tipsy. That's how my friends like me." This is rarely true – most people on drink simply become louder and more incoherent. You can be just as funny and likeable sober but you will probably judge yourself more. Allow yourself to be childish and uninhibited on occasions without having your Parent staring disapprovingly at you from within.

Drinking **to feel less inhibited** – "I'd be far too shy going on a date or joining in if I didn't have a drink in my hand." Take some time before your date or evening out to build your confidence in other ways. Look in the mirror and tell yourself that you look good and feel good and are going to have a good time. If you get tipsy or drunk, you won't be able to assess if your date is a good match or not, and you may even put yourself at risk. Ask yourself if alcohol had a negative effect in your previous relationships.

▨ Drinking because of **peer group pressure** – "I was going to go home but it was my round and if I didn't buy it – and have one too – I'd be called a skinflint." Soft drinks or sodas can cost almost as much as alcoholic drinks these days, so there is no reason not to keep buying your round.

▨ Drinking **to be intimate** – "My partner and I always drink wine before every sexual encounter as part of our ritual for intimacy and relaxation." You and your partner may want to think about the reasons why you feel like being tipsy or even drunk to have sex. Is it something you both feel you need, or just one of you, who then feels more confident and loosens up? It's a good thing for a couple to be able to talk about such matters and to try having sex without the booze. You may be surprised by the outcome: too much alcohol dulls the senses, so the experience might be even more exciting and sensual. Plus, losing weight by not drinking so much will ultimately make you feel even more confident and sexy.

Most of my clients tell me that it would be easier for them to stop drinking completely than to try to limit their consumption. That's fine if that's how you feel, but my concern with such a drastic decision is that you may not be able to stick to it in the long term. Instead, I would encourage you to learn to drink more mindfully. As with eating, nothing is forbidden.

You just have to stop when you have had enough.

First of all, it is important to assess how much you drink on a weekly basis, which is where the Food and Emotions Diary becomes so useful again. It is too easy to forget to count our drinks, both by their number and by the quantity in each glass. Writing it down in the moment will give you a much more realistic view. You might record that you had a glass of wine, but how big was it? A large glass holds twice the amount of wine compared to a small one, for example.

Drinking and calories

Here is a quick approximate calorie count of some of the drinks you might have regularly:

- Standard glass of wine (175ml/6fl oz) – 159 calories

- Pint of beer (568ml/20fl oz) – 182 calories

- Bottle of lager (330ml/11fl oz) – 142 calories

- Single spirit (25ml/1fl oz) – 61 calories

- Alcopop/alcoholic soda (275ml/9½fl oz) – 170 calories

- Pint of cider (568ml/20fl oz) – 239 calories

- Glass of prosecco/champagne (125ml/4fl oz) – 89 calories

(Drinkaware UK)

This means that one night out a week can quickly add up to a lot of extra calories over the year, especially if we do little to burn it up. Tot up your own calorie and unit count from your Food and

Emotions Diary and see what it comes to. Write it down. You may be shocked.

The extra weight we gain from drinking doesn't just come from the fermented sugars in the alcohol. There are other, often unforeseen, consequences. After a few drinks (two or three large glasses of wine or pints of beer), hunger kicks in and a chemical reaction caused by a decrease in our blood glucose levels leads us to crave foods high in fat or carbohydrates, adding massively to our calorie intake.

Not to mention what you ate or drank earlier that day, or the cooked breakfast you feel like eating in the morning to get over your hangover.

I know the thought of totting up all these calories may sound boring or even fussy, and you might even start to feel nervous at this point because you've done all this before on diets and it hasn't worked. The difference now is that I am not here to tell you to stop drinking, just as I am not here to tell you to stop eating. You are the Adult, who bought this book because you wanted things to change. To make those changes, first analyse the situation and then you can take the decisions you feel suit you best. You may think that drinking gives you some kind of freedom from the anxieties of your life, but where is the freedom in being wracked with guilt or overcome with shame each time you get drunk?

"I had no idea how out of control my drinking had become until I started to add up how much I was consuming. Not only was I appalled by the extra 4,000 or so calories a week my drinking was piling on, but I realized that I was a borderline alcoholic and that really scared me."

Issues with alcohol

Drinkaware UK defines alcoholism as "a strong, often uncontrollable, desire to drink". Those who are considered to be alcoholics often place their need for a drink above all other obligations, including work and family, and may build up a physical tolerance and/or experience withdrawal symptoms if they stop. The definition of "harmful drinking" is a random pattern of drinking which can damage your health. One such example might be binge drinking and getting into a fight or falling over. This kind of drinking may well develop into full-blown alcoholism if it becomes a regular habit.

ARE YOU AN ALCOHOLIC?

Someone is considered to be an alcoholic if they show any of the following signs on a regular basis:

- developing such a tolerance to alcohol that they need to drink more to get drunk

- drinking larger amounts for longer periods on a regular basis

- becoming obsessive about getting and consuming alcohol

- falling down on their responsibilities at home or work

- missing out on important events in order to drink, or because of their drinking

- having an inability to give up drinking even when it has catastrophic consequences.

Physical symptoms may include an increased heart rate, anxiety, sweating, trembling, nausea and/or vomiting, hallucinations, insomnia and seizures that can be fatal. Whether someone is suffering from full-blown alcoholism or not, alcohol-related liver disease has risen massively in many Western societies and doesn't usually cause any symptoms until the damage has been done. This means that many people don't even know that they're at risk, or appreciate that their excessive drinking can lead to cancer.

The liver is a vital organ for our health that can be adversely affected by alcohol, obesity, diabetes and hepatitis C – all of which are on the rise as well. Recent reports have estimated that the incidence of chronic liver disease, liver cancer and cirrhosis in the "baby boomer" generation has risen dramatically, as has the occurence of liver cancer in young people. It is also more likely to affect men than women. These kinds of figures and their impact on the health services and on people's lives have led to initiatives for minimum pricing of alcohol, but the problem isn't being solved.

To avoid becoming one of those statistics, we each have to make some choices about what we drink, and how much. It will help to answer the following questions, in total honesty. Remember, no one will read your answers but you:

1. At what age did you first start drinking?

2. Do you feel that you drink normally?

3. Do you ever drink specifically to get drunk or to "drown your sorrows"?

4. Do you have a reputation as a drinker that you feel you benefit from?

5. Do you drink to feel better or to function better in some way?

6. Do you ever drink in the mornings?

7. Do you ever drink alone to avoid feeling lonely or to numb your emotions?

8. Do you ever feel guilty about your drinking?

9. How often do you drink? Daily? Three times a week? Only at weekends?

10. Do you regularly stop drinking for any period of time, such as "Dry January", or for a few days per week?

11. If you stop, do you suffer any withdrawal symptoms or do you feel healthier?

12. Do you ever engage in binge drinking (more than five drinks per session)? If so, how often?

13. Using your Food and Emotions Diary, add up how many drinks you had in an average week. How many days did you have more than three drinks?

14. Have you ever passed out because of drink? If so, when was the last time?

15. Do you ever suffer from memory loss or have difficulty speaking when drinking?

16. Have you ever got into a fight or some other trouble, or had an accident while drinking? Have you or anyone else been injured because of your drinking?

17. Have you ever been arrested for drink driving?

18. Has drinking ever caused you any difficulties in a relationship?

19. Have you ever resolved to stop drinking for a period but been unable to keep it up?

20. Have you ever sought professional or other help about your drinking?

21. Is there a history of alcohol problems in your family?

After you have written down your answers, read through them carefully and see if there are any patterns emerging. If, for example, you have got into trouble through drinking on more than one occasion, summon up that experience and remember how bad you felt afterward. Reformed alcoholics often say, "Bad things didn't always happen every time I drank, but every time a bad thing happened drink was involved." If that is true of you too, then now may be the time to address the problem before it gets out of control.

What about your relationships? Everyone has arguments with those they live or work with, but when people are drunk they tend to lose their inhibitions and say and do things that they may regret later. Most domestic abuse callouts attended by the emergency services prove to be fuelled by alcohol or drugs. The same goes for vandalism and other violence.

Binge drinking (like binge eating) can be especially damaging to our health and lead to all kinds of other problems. Those under the influence can become vulnerable to physical attack. Drinkers can be quick to anger and get into fights more easily. This kind of drinking is almost always social and often ends up with unhealthy late-night eating, which can undermine plans to lose weight and lead a healthier life.

Flag up the times and places that you felt most susceptible to drinking too much and think about how you can address similar occasions in the future.

"My dad drank too much and that ended up causing the split from my mum. I vowed I'd never be like him and I'm not – apart from the times when I become an idiot in the pub with my mates. All my willpower flies out the window, and the next morning I feel guilty and hungover and sick to my stomach in every way."

Once a client realizes that he or she needs to address their drinking, they ask me to set them some rules. People like rules because then they don't have to think about things too deeply.

■ "Should I only drink on the weekend, or every two days?"

■ "Is it okay if I only drink on a night out?"

■ "What if I stop drinking at home?"

I can't give them an answer because those kinds of rules sound too much like an alcohol diet to me.

You will know by now that diets are not my thing.

The problem is that we humans often feel safer when we have rules, which is just as well because there are rules everywhere: when we drive, when we interact with others, where we smoke, what we do at work, as parents, as residents, as commuters. We are constantly being told what we should do, where we should go, how we should lead our lives, even how we should sort our waste products. All day long, all year long, our life is dominated by rules that have been created to make our society safe and viable. Although most of them are sensible and necessary, we can feel at times that our freedom is slowly shrinking.

Whenever we get tipsy or drunk we can feel as if we are somehow regaining that freedom. We are suddenly free to express ourselves the way we want – free to be silly, to laugh at stupid things, free to be more authentically ourselves. If we have adopted the Parent ego state in order to obey all the rules, when we drink it is replaced by our rebellious Child who quickly reappears and wants to smash them.

What we have to learn and understand is that there are other ways to be authentic. Alcohol works only for a very short period of time and then the shame and guilt kicks in. Before we know it, our Parent ego reminds us why we should stick to the rules in the first place. The more you are authentic to yourself and to others, the less you will need alcohol to soften those rules. You will stop seeing them within the non-stop Parent–Child conversation in your head and view them instead with Adult eyes that help you see that the rules are really designed to allow you to live more freely and authentically.

For example, the unwritten social rule that it isn't fair to make too much noise at night and disturb your neighbours means that you, too, can enjoy the peace of your own home each night to recover from your day. The regulation governing drinking and driving is to keep you and others safe. The edicts not to spit in the streets or smoke in restaurants are to stop us offending anyone or causing them any harm. A decision to raise the price of alcohol and cigarettes is designed to help us help ourselves.

If you are more comfortable living by rules, then by all means create your own when it comes to your drinking. You probably have them already but didn't even realize it – for example the unwritten (and often subconscious) rule that you will undoubtedly drink alcohol when you are on a night out with family or friends. This is a rule created by habit and custom, fed by anticipation and expectation.

Now you can make up a new rule for yourself. Before going out with the intention to drink all night, prepare yourself for another scenario – a positive rather than a negative one. Without stressing about it, stop and take a minute or two to reconsider your plans. Think about the reasons behind this "decision" to drink and consider if it's really worth the calories and the headache, instead of doing it almost as a reflex.

It may be Friday and you may be going out with your friends because that is what happens every week, but it doesn't mean you have to drink excessively. Don't be over-judgmental. Have an Adult-to-Adult conversation with yourself. All of this shouldn't take more than a minute or two, but it will make a massive difference to the outcome of your evening.

Ask yourself the following questions:

- Will your night be more fun if you get tipsy or drunk? Will it really make any difference if you don't? And if so, will this difference be positive or negative?

- How much money will you spend buying alcoholic drinks? How much would you save if you didn't?

- Is having too many drinks worth sabotaging your weight-loss plan, when it has been going so well?

- Are you more likely to make unhealthy eating choices when you drink too much?

- How will you feel about that tomorrow? Will you have a hangover and/or be wracked with guilt?

- Will drinking too much affect your sleep? Will this have an adverse effect on your eating tomorrow too?

Remember, I am not trying to take away your short-term pleasure with this advice; my intention is to add to your longterm sense of wellbeing and contentment once you achieve your goal. The idea is not to be stone cold sober but to drink moderately by being more mindful. Then when you get to the place where you are going to spend your evening, employ these few tips to help you achieve that:

- Decide that you will have only two alcoholic drinks and intersperse these with soft drinks or sodas. Maybe leave your credit card at home or take only enough cash to cover that many drinks (and/or to buy your fair share of rounds).

- Consider telling your most trusted, intimate friends what you are trying to do and asking for their help, but not in a way that makes them jointly responsible for your commitment.

- Don't start drinking alcohol straight away, wait for the second or third round. We usually drink faster at first because we think it helps us connect and "settle in". Make your first couple of drinks sparkling water or something else soft and refreshing.

- If you feel peer group pressure to make sure you buy a round, then buy the first round (which will be cheaper anyway if you order just a tonic instead of a gin and tonic) and the next round you have to pay for will take longer to come around.

- Once you do start drinking, be sure to order smaller drinks (half-pints, single shots).

- Make sure that you drink plenty of water to quench your thirst and are drinking alcohol only for the taste, not because you are thirsty.

As with the Food and Emotions Diary, ask yourself how you're feeling during the evening, being sure to take deep breaths to connect to your emotions. Are you tired? Are you having fun? Do you feel like staying longer, or would you rather head back home? Do you like the conversations you're having? Are you being authentically yourself?

Research shows that we only truly appreciate our first two drinks before the pleasure of the taste diminishes. So, on round three, ask yourself, are you still enjoying your drink? If not, why sacrifice your weight-loss project and waste more money on something you're not even appreciating?

Is everybody else's drunkenness becoming boring? Are they becoming loud and incoherent? Why not slip out of the door and go home before they even notice?

> **"One morning I woke up with a terrible headache in some stranger's bed and I didn't even know who he was. I felt disgusted with myself. That's when I knew I had to stop drinking so much."**

Very often your body tells you, "I've had enough," but you're somehow disconnected and you just keep on drinking, which can quickly get out of hand. Only by trying to follow your new rules can you discover that drinking moderately can be extremely pleasurable. You enjoy sharing the moment with others, you choose to drink something you like and, afterward, you still feel great about yourself.

If none of this seems feasible to you and isn't part of your usual pattern, then you probably won't buy what I'm saying. This is because you are resistant to change, and change can be scary if it means facing the unknown.

You may worry that you will lose friends if you follow my suggestions and stop drinking so much socially or duck out of the evening earlier than usual. You may be anxious that they will think you are being mean about buying your round, or boring. You think they'll imagine that you are abandoning them by not participating so enthusiastically. But if some of your "friends" think you're not worth being with just because you are drinking less in order to lead a happier, healthier life, then maybe you should start to question those friendships.

To be able to see the obvious benefits of moderate drinking, you have to be able to project yourself into the near future: you will sleep better, you will make wiser food choices, you won't be hungover, and you will have more money to spend on other things. Imagine all of that and then think how pleasurable it will be to celebrate the new you with those you love and who love you.

TO RECAP

- Alcohol is ubiquitous, so accept that the temptation will always be there and develop sensible strategies to deal with it.

- If drinking is something you do out of habit to take the edge off your day, think of other ways to do that – going for a run, having a bath, being with your family.

- Become better informed about the damaging effects of alcohol on your body and think of the long-term consequences for your health and your weight.

- Add up your calorie count from alcohol, the number of units you are consuming, and the amount of money you are spending to remind you of the overall costs to your health, weight and pocket.

- Answer the questionnaire about your drinking and look for patterns and bad habits. If you feel you have a problem, then seek professional help (see page 265).

- Devise new rules for yourself in preparation for any event at which you might be tempted to drink or eat too much.

- Be authentically yourself and stop worrying so much about what others might think of you. Remember, these fears might sabotage your weight loss. By addressing them, you can change.

- Make your reduction in alcohol intake part of your conscious decision to lead a healthier, happier life and not to overload your body with toxins.

CASE STUDY

Nicole came to see me two years ago because she was managing her weight in a way that wasn't sustainable and was slowly losing control. Over the course of the previous four years she had gained 6 kilos (1 stone) in weight and, because she was very self-conscious, her anxiety around her body image was growing.

She was a 39-year-old single woman working as a manager for an estate agent. She worked hard and she played hard. She said she wanted "the best of everything". Describing herself as a party girl, she enjoyed her nights out with girlfriends and her occasional dates. Her way to manage her weight had been by careful calorie-counting but she loved to drink and get "tipsy" two or three times a week, so to factor in the extra calories on the days she was planning to drink, she would eat one small meal at lunchtime and nothing else.

Her maths were simple. In a drastic and prohibitive way, she swapped some of her calorie allowance for the day with those she'd consume in alcohol. Similarly, whenever she knew she was going to an event where she felt she had to eat she wouldn't eat the day before. The funny thing is that her friends knew about it; she didn't make a secret of it and they sometimes praised her for her willpower.

Then her system started slowly weakening and the weight started to climb. She made a few drastic attempts to get back on track, not eating for up to two days at a time, but things got out of control and this was very scary for her.

She had put so much effort and energy into managing her weight that she felt powerless now that her system had stopped working.

By the time she came to see me, she was frightened of changing her pattern as she was convinced it worked and had no faith in any other. It took Nicole three sessions before she could accept that she would have to reconsider her eating habits, but we eventually got there. In the first two weeks she did put on a few pounds, as she was finding it difficult to moderate her drinking. She complained bitterly to me about that - "I'm paying you to lose weight and look what's happening!" I wasn't concerned, as I knew it would take a bit of time for her to find the right balance after so many years on her unhealthy system. Within five weeks she was on track and it took her altogether three months to lose the weight she'd put on in recent years. She was so over the moon that she cried, "I'm free like I've never been before!" at the end of our final session. I saw her again recently by chance and she had never looked better.

8

EMBRACE THE REAL YOU

"Being thin again made me feel completely differently about myself and about the way others treated me. I realized that if I could lose all that weight, I could do anything, and that included cutting out those who weren't really on my side."

By the final chapter, most diet books simply sign off and leave you to embark on yet another yo-yo experience of success followed by the inevitable failure. The authors rarely remind you that the weight that took years to put on won't just drop away instantly. It will take time and patience, plus a serious evaluation of the root causes of your overeating.

Congratulations on getting this far and for understanding that there is another way. We live in a world where people want quick solutions, so I applaud you for sticking with me and allowing me to help you find a better way and make peace with your true self. Bravo!

There may, of course, be times along the way when you find that the process isn't working as well as you hoped, or something may happen to sabotage you. That is completely normal. I see it very often with my clients and half-expect it with many.

"I got angry with my mum/dad/sister/partner/child and ended up drinking too much and eating an entire pizza!" one might complain. Or, "My life is just too busy. I'll never be able to maintain this level of mindfulness about what I buy, cook and eat!"

One or two lapses like this will never be enough to throw you off message completely, but they will be indicative of the kind of fear you may experience as you start to face up to your emotions and appreciate that this isn't as simple as just cutting down on calories. If, for instance, you binge eat whenever you are in the company of someone toxic, by looking at your Food and Emotions Diary and seeing that pattern for the first time you will realize that you have to address the problems with that relationship, or at least your emotional reaction to it.

Change is almost always scary. It takes us out of our comfort zone. The quickest way to sabotage yourself is to give in to the fears and let things stay the way they are, continually overeating to quash your emotions or compensate for something. It is time to face up to reality.

Remember that maintaining the status quo isn't what you want – or you would never have picked up this book to begin with, hopeful of a whole new approach that would take you to a better place than the one you are trapped in now.

The other thing that most diet books fail to address is what happens once you reach your ideal weight.

We often think that once we are slim life will suddenly become so much easier and we will finally be happy.

We need to ask ourselves the following questions:

- Will my life be easier if I lose weight?

- What if it isn't?

- Will my new body feel just like I hoped it would?

- Will I be satisfied with my reflection in the mirror?

- What will my weight loss alter in my life?

- Perhaps more importantly, what won't it have changed?

- What will it be like to be slim?

- Am I prepared to be the real me at last?

As long as I have done my job right, by the end of your weight-loss project you should be free of worry about your size or shape, and be embracing the many changes to both your habits and your beliefs that you have brought about.

The chief one will be the realization that there is another way to live your life and that things are not always predetermined. All your preconceptions about fad diets and dieting will have been thrown out of the window.

You don't have to stay stuck in a rut or stick to a repetitive pattern of non-mindful behaviour and eating. You can finally stop waiting for someone or something to "save" you but instead take responsibility for yourself.

The choice to change is yours, and yours alone.

This is a crucial moment for self-reflection and the chance to cement lasting change.

> **"I'm a successful adult but often felt like a naughty child. It took me ages to realize that the bad habits I'd inherited from my parents – who'd lived through a war and had their own reasons for drinking too much and eating unhealthily – were things I could change if I put my mind to it. When I did, I finally felt like a grown-up."**

It is my responsibility as your therapist to help you through the many and varied emotions you might be feeling by the end of your weight-loss project. My focus won't be on whether you've lost all the kilos or pounds you wanted or got down to the size you were when you were last truly content, it will be on getting you to the point where you are happy enough with yourself so that it's no longer a worry.

By then I would expect you to be enjoying eating food only when you are really hungry and no longer overeating to compensate for the unhappiness, fear, loneliness or anger in your life because you will have found other, healthier ways to manage these.

I would also urge you to move your body more – right from the start. "Oh God," I can hear some moan, "Philippe's going to tell me to join a gym!" No, I'm not. I know they work for some people but personally I hate them, especially the kind where everyone looks at everyone else in the (usually deeply unflattering) wall-to-wall mirrors. Nor do I see the appeal of running on a treadmill every night when you feel as if you have already been running on a treadmill all day. What's wrong with the great outdoors?

Getting away from our home or work environment is one of the best things we can do for our mental health. It takes us out of ourselves and occupies our mind, replacing the usual worries which take up so much room. Once we rid ourselves of all that worry and stop checking our reflection in shop windows, touching our own bodies constantly to see if we are "fat or thin" that day, or thinking about food three hundred times a day, we need to have a plan to fill that time and space with something else. Now is the time to move forward, to be more active and proactive. I can't think of a better plan than exercise, which has so many other benefits too. So here are some tips for getting more:

- Choose something you really enjoy – I play badminton but I also like to walk and cycle. Many of my clients love Zumba and other dance-related classes. Others play sports.

- Pick something that involves socializing and isn't solitary like solo running. This way you have the added advantage of the endorphins that are released when we have fun.

- Select something that's within your budget – hundreds of thousands of pounds are lost each year on unused gym memberships that are often very expensive, only piling on the guilt and anxiety when you don't go. So much else is free and right on your doorstep.

- Find something local and convenient. The best flamenco class might be five bus stops and a ten-minute walk away but that won't be so much fun on dark winter nights, so pick a class or an activity that fits in better with your way of life.

- Go with a friend. This will give you extra motivation to keep doing it and not duck out when you don't feel like it or would prefer to be a couch potato. Remember not to make your friend responsible if you stop after they decide to drop out. Take your own responsibility!

- Try to do something that regularly makes you breathless – connect to your own body sensations of sweat, muscle and bone. Something like yoga is fine – or choose something else if you feel you would benefit more from a team activity.

- Find something that helps others in your community as much as it helps you – offer to coach a junior football team, volunteer to do some gardening for an elderly neighbour, take someone underprivileged to a park or an exercise class, or go play table tennis at a homeless shelter. Helping others produces so many feel-good chemicals in our bodies that – if we can combine it with more exercise – it is a win-win situation for everyone.

- Savour the changes in your body as you continue to exercise. Take pleasure in your new muscle definition and your looser clothing. Celebrate the differences you are making to your life.

> **"My girlfriend and I joined a laughter yoga class that basically involved laughing for ninety minutes once a week. Our teacher described it as "internal jogging". Although it felt strange at first, we soon got the hang of it and running around, clapping our hands, or wriggling our bodies while laughing out loud turned out to be the greatest fun we've had in years."**

Change can be painful for some people. But remember, it will never be as painful as being stuck on a treadmill of yo-yo dieting and self-loathing.

For some people, a change in the shape and size of their bodies can spark a desire for radical change in other areas of their lives too. If, for example, when analysing your Food and Emotions Diary you realize that you have mostly eaten unhealthily at work because you are bored and unhappy with your job, then you might decide to change that job or to fill your life outside work with something so satisfying and fulfilling that the job no longer plays such a major role in your life.

If you see that you are involved with someone who is encouraging or enabling your bad habits (probably because of that person's own fears about change), you may feel the need to get out of that relationship. If you accept that you are predominantly lonely (whether alone or not), you might develop a whole new perspective and think about embarking on a completely different way of life in which you feel more connected to others.

As a therapist, it is my role to make sure that those decisions are coming from a safe, secure place and aren't part of a new obsession. Many people tend to swap one addiction for another, and that isn't healthy either. It is important to remember that not everything we've learned from the previous chapters means that our life has to change in every way if we are to have the body that we want. We will, of course, have to make some empowering, liberating adjustments, but it's not about revolution.

Once you make the changes that are best for you, then you can see how that impacts on other aspects of your life. Good news travels fast and the people that matter in your life will generally be happy for you. They may even surprise you with their reactions when, inspired by your achievements, they choose to make similar changes in their own lives.

Give yourself permission to make mistakes and – if that happens – regard them as an experiment; a learning experience. If one of your changes doesn't work for you, don't consider the attempt as a failure but congratulate yourself for having tried and take time to figure out what would suit you better.

Another unexpected issue with weight loss is how others react to us once we're slim. After I lost all my weight I can remember people telling me repeatedly, "Philippe, you look fantastic!" They might even say, "You look so much better than when I last saw you." It astonished me that my weight and the way I looked could be a topic for so much discussion, especially among people I wasn't intimate with at all and who I'd never expected to comment on my appearance. It had been something I'd been dealing with in silence, and suddenly people were openly commenting on my size and shape.

Then the inevitable question followed: "But how did you do it?" Or perhaps, "Come on, tell me which diet you've been on." Unlike most people who are on a diet who tell everyone around them about it ad nauseam, only those closest to me knew that I was living a different kind of life and eating more healthily. I recommend you do the same too, because this process is so much more personal than just a weight-loss programme. You will be changing so much more than your weight.

Naturally, everyone else who saw the evidence of my success wanted to know which diet I had been on so they could try it too.

I lost so much weight that some of my friends even believed I had undergone surgery for stomach stapling. They probably still do (I didn't, of course).

"I've been eating less," I'd reply simply. "Yes, I exercised more and I was far more careful about when and what I ate and drank." If pressed, I might add, "I also learned how to manage my stress differently and I listened to what my body was telling me. I was able to differentiate between my genuine hunger and what my brain was dealing with emotionally."

"So, what exactly did you do?" they'd persist, "Give up drink? Join a gym? Do you still eat desserts? You've always loved your desserts!"

"Yes, I eat desserts sometimes, if I feel like it."

"Was it very hard?"

"No," I replied honestly. "Being fat was hard."

I didn't feel the need to explain any further, and neither will you.

Each time anyone tried to keep on digging about how much I'd lost and through what method, it took me back to my own therapy when I was so much heavier, and this frustrated me. I didn't want to be reminded of that period, because even before I lost all the weight I'd already changed something about my life and moved on. I just had to smile and politely thank them.

Then I got to a point I'd never expected, with people telling me to stop losing any more. "Are you all right? Have you been ill?" some asked, especially if they hadn't seen me for a while or weren't aware that I was losing weight. Others would assure me, "But you look so much older!" or warn, "If you lose much more, you'll go all wrinkly," as if they had the right to tell me how much I should lose. It is true that people who lose a lot of weight can sometimes look a little older at first, but it's important to remember that your body age will probably be years younger once you are healthy and no longer binge eating.

"People were different around me once I lost weight. They were more respectful in some way – almost shy. It was as if I was someone else and not the person they knew and loved. They seemed a little wary. It took a bit of time to make them see that I was still the same old me."

Another problem for me was the responses of friends who used to enjoy watching me eat everything they'd prepared for me. Seeing me leave food on my plate or not ask for a second helping upset them and they couldn't understand why I no longer devoured everything in sight. "What's wrong, Philippe? Don't you like the food?" they'd ask, with sad faces. "Aren't you having fun?" Their expressions made me realize that they missed the old me, the big man who had created an entire persona around eating and living high on the hog.

That then also threw up lots of questions about how much room my weight and my eating habits had previously taken up in our relationship. For some, the fact that I no longer finished everything up also left them with a personal dilemma, because they suddenly had leftovers that challenged their own eating issues.

These kinds of reactions are not uncommon, and many of my clients experience unforeseen anxieties sparked by others. I worked with one woman whose marriage broke up after she lost 25 kilos (4 stone). Her therapy proved to her that her husband had secretly enjoyed taking the moral high ground over her weight issues and felt threatened by her new sexual attractiveness. It became clear to them both that he didn't really want her to succeed, and that raised all sorts of problems between them that couldn't easily be addressed. The issues had always been there, but it took her weight loss to finally expose them.

We now know from Chapter 5 that we all live within systems or networks and are influenced by those around us. The ripple effect of others' comments and behaviours can impact negatively on our resolve to lose weight and live more healthily. If this is something you face while losing weight, then it would be a good time to revisit that chapter and remind yourself how Systemic Therapy helps us deal with such issues and not use them as a means of self-sabotage (see page 105).

In my own case I am pleased to report that I didn't lose a single friend either during the process or after, and that is the case for most people. Once they had got over the novelty of seeing me slim, they were all fantastically supportive. So be prepared for the changes you make to affect your relationships with others, but don't worry about how much. Since none of these changes happen overnight, you will be able to manage them all with serenity and confidence.

> **"My boss has always been very passive-aggressive and every time she had a go at me in the past I'd automatically reach for the chocolate. Now that I know how to manage her and the stress and anxiety she creates, I step outside and sit in the garden for five minutes to calm down. It feels like a little victory over her, plus it saves me from eating a bar of milk chocolate every day."**

Several of my clients have believed that when they lost weight all their problems would melt away, but that isn't realistic. Problems will undoubtedly still exist, but you will be happier and far better able to cope with them without automatically turning to food or drink for comfort.

Others expect to look in the mirror after they have lost weight and see the younger person they had in their minds when they came up with their ideal size. Instead, they see someone much older, with the "scars" of life on their faces and bodies – just like the rest of us. Losing a lot of weight (and by that I mean more than a few kilos or pounds) can leave us with flabby tummies, stretch marks, wrinkles and excess skin. I know because I have all of the above. It is a shame when it happens, because we have made so much effort and taken so much time to get to the point where we are happy with our bodies, and yet every day we can still see signs that remind us that we were once overweight. These physical scars can sometimes reawaken emotional ones.

In this instance, I ask my clients, "Do you like how you look now?" They nod but often add, "Yes, except when I'm undressed." I ask them what they mean, and they tell me that they hate the way their body sags in certain places, or how it looks in a bathing suit. Some of them opt for cosmetic surgery to make them feel better. I don't encourage it, but that is their choice.

I also remind them that they can improve their skin and general appearance in all sorts of ways that don't involve surgery, and suggest they indulge themselves if they feel like it. They'll be saving so much money since they changed their drinking and eating habits that they can not only afford it, but deserve it too.

For those like me that don't want surgery, I remind them that they have come such a long way on their journey to better health and happiness that the truth is these things don't matter so much anymore. They have changed in so many other ways and with such positive results for their physical and mental wellbeing that they're finally able to accept their minor blemishes or how they look naked, both of which are worth the price of the fantastic results they have achieved.

Another question I am very often asked is, "Once I've reached my target weight, will I have to focus on eating healthily for the rest of my life if I want to keep the weight off?"

The answer to the question is yes, most of the time you will have to focus on eating healthily, but not in a way that will be anything but pleasurable. Although this answer may seem daunting at first, or may even be enough to put some off trying in the first place, it has a positive flip side that you probably haven't considered.

Sure, there can be a sense that after years of being trapped in a body you hated, once you lose all the weight you wanted you will simply be trapped in a new way of life that could be just as demanding. What you have to ask yourself is which of the two "traps" you would prefer – the one where you were secretly miserable and probably hiding your unhealthy eating habits from all those around you while you wasted hours every day obsessing about food, or the one where you look forward to shopping, preparing, cooking and eating something that is good for you and for all those within your networks?

In time, you will realize that even though it isn't always easy to change your habits, it's not that difficult to maintain them once you have achieved this new way of thinking. This is especially true because by eating more mindfully you will instil these new patterns deeply in you – and maybe even help those around you too. And don't forget that this is not a restrictive diet. There is no taboo food. It is all about having the right balance throughout the week.

Best of all, you will also have more energy, and your rebuilt self-confidence will take you to a happier place psychologically. And contrary to what many people believe, overeating and being overweight is not an easy way of life by any means. It isn't an option you have chosen because it's the one that requires less control, as we can see throughout this book. It is by far more demanding in many ways than eating mindfully and healthily.

"I was worried that I'd have to be careful about my eating and drinking for the rest of my life after I lost all my weight but it didn't feel like that at all. Just as I don't worry about having to brush my teeth or check my makeup, my new patterns of eating and drinking became completely natural to me and it was so liberating not to have to even think about them."

TO RECAP

- Congratulations on getting this far. Don't think that this is where the hard work really begins, because it's been hard before, maybe for your whole life.

- Be prepared for lapses and self-sabotage. Changing your eating and drinking habits is not a straight path.

- Remember that although change is scary it is better than what went before.

- Face up to reality. There has never been a better time to do this and change your life.

- Accept that not everything will be better once you lose weight.

- Prepare yourself for unforeseen consequences.

- Move your body more in a social, fun way.

- Change doesn't always mean revolution, so think carefully before making further radical changes.

- Be prepared for people's reactions to your weight loss, not all of which will be good.

- Think about what you are going to tell people about how you managed it.

- Expect physical changes that may not be as you imagined.

- Accept that your choices to be healthier and happier are now a lifelong commitment.

- Enjoy your new energy and self-confidence, and remember that being unhealthy took up far more time and energy than being healthy does.

In this final chapter I have not one but three case studies for you, including one about me, that I think perfectly sum up the ethos of this book and how you can use the tools I have provided you with to deal with your own challenges in the future.

Read them through carefully and see how the different coping strategies can be adopted for different situations and free you to have the body you are comfortable with. There is no magic wand. Most of this is common sense, but as Voltaire once said, "Common sense is not so common." Sometimes it takes someone else to point it out.

CASE STUDY 1

Cassandra is 44 and works from home as a "virtual" personal assistant. She has a good job, a great social life and, although single, is enjoying her freedom. Working from home is a new experience for her and, although she likes the flexibility it gives her, she wasn't prepared for how solitary it made her feel. Unlike in a busy office, her apartment was very quiet and there was no one to interact directly with.

Whenever she needed a screen break, she would put the kettle on to make herself a cup of tea and invariably rummage through the cupboard or the fridge for something to eat. After 18 months of this she had gained almost 10 kilos (a stone and a half) and was unhappy with her shape. As her working environment wasn't going to change, she knew that she had to change something within it and so she came to see me. After discussing the various options open to her, she decided to visit an animal shelter with a friend and they each rescued a stray dog. Hers was a loving two-year-old Staffordshire terrier named Dolly.

Having a dog gave Cassandra a reason to get up from her desk and move her body more often. She would walk it in the local park at least twice a day, often with her friend and his new dog, or on her own. She found that having a dog created an instant connection with other dog owners, many of whom she met frequently and one of whom she soon started dating.

By the time she lost all her weight she felt healthier, happier and less lonely. She had found something positive to fill the space that food used to occupy in her life. Now, when people asked her how she had lost the weight, she told them truthfully that getting a dog had been a key factor and they accepted that.

By the way, I am happy to report that Dolly lost 4 kilos (9 pounds) too!

CASE STUDY 2

Christopher, 44, lives in a busy city where he is the well-paid district manager of one of the largest supermarket chains. He is divorced and childless, living in his own home, and enjoys a life that is full but not very stressful. He is very happy with his girlfriend, with whom he goes on regular weekend hikes.

Despite all appearances, he often feels a kind of "emptiness", as if something is lacking in his life. He then feels guilty for thinking that when he has such a comfortable life. His parents and two brothers work much harder than he does for less recognition – both financial and social – and he feels guilty about this too, imagining that they and others must think he has been able to succeed without much effort. He cannot accept that his position was earned through his own dedication, talent and excellent managerial skills.

In recent years, he has gained about 10 kilos (a stone and a half) and he blamed his easy access to processed food for that, but after some analysis we quickly realized that this was not the case. He was eating to fill the emptiness inside him. Paradoxically, by gaining weight this emptiness was only accentuated because it increased his poor self-image of unworthiness and idleness.

I suggested that Christopher take on some charitable work with the underprivileged for a few hours a week, depending on his availability. I thought this would have the double benefit of making him feel more fulfilled and reminding him of his own blessings. He immediately liked the idea and considered which causes were closest to his heart. Having investigated the subject, and because he often saw vagrants hanging around outside the supermarkets he visited, he joined a charity that helps homeless people.

It was gratifying how quickly this activity benefited him. He immersed himself in the charity and used his people skills to make good connections with staff and the homeless, forging deep ties. He even went beyond his mission by bringing unsold food from the supermarkets to the charity kitchen as often as possible, and going on sponsored hikes with his girlfriend to raise money for his new friends. His weight problems are far behind him now that his life has become so much more meaningful. He recently said to me, "I haven't been on a food diet. I've been on a heart diet."

CASE STUDY 3

It has been nearly 20 years since I lost all the weight I gained while I was married and living in Belgium. Many of my clients ask me how I manage that after so many years. The answer is confidence.

There are, of course, occasions when I continue to eat when I'm no longer hungry, but any time it's happened it has never been to the same degree that it used to be and I don't now feel bad or blame myself as I used to. My Parent state of mind comes into play to help me understand what happened. I ask myself, was I stressed or tired? Did the company I was in have any influence? Was I trying to please someone? Now that I have been doing this for so long, the answer comes quite quickly and I am able to see how to address it.

It happened to me again not so long ago when I was going to a picnic organized by some very good friends of mine. I was taking a friend with me who I really appreciate, but who doesn't always feel confident in the company of strangers.

Once we arrived she put on a happy face but I could feel her anxiety rising, which only added to mine. I tried to stay by her side and reassure her but it wasn't really helpful. I was feeling both concerned for her and upset at not being able to have as much fun as I'd hoped with my friends, as I had been looking forward to the event all week. I ate and drank more than I needed and I was aware that I wasn't being mindful, but it didn't stop me.

The two of us left the picnic earlier than most of the others and headed home separately. Back in my apartment I thought to myself, "Well, that's interesting. How and why did those circumstances make me drink and eat too much?" I wasn't concerned about the weight because I knew I'd balance that out in the next few days. But I wanted to make sure I wouldn't put myself through such an uncomfortable experience again, or at least that I'd manage it in a different way.

I considered what my options had been before and during the picnic. I'd known in advance that my friend wouldn't be comfortable there, so I could have decided not to invite her. I could have left with her sooner and gone back on my own, or I could have suggested that if she wasn't having much fun then she was free to duck out of the day. Perhaps most importantly of all, I could have spent less time fussing over her and worrying how she was feeling and enjoyed my friends as I intended.

What I had done instead was to blame her in some way, making her responsible for my overeating, which wasn't fair or right. She didn't put that food in my mouth, and nor did she force me to drink all that wine. I realized that at the picnic I was dealing with two things: a woman whose anxiety in many ways reminded me of my mother, and my irrepressible desire to be with my friends. That was too much to handle in one afternoon!

I remembered that my friend told me several times, "I'm fine, Philippe. Go and chat with your friends," but I felt guilty. Meanwhile, my friends were all telling me how good it was to see me and my resentment was growing. I was on a mission I knew only too well – trying to please everyone, something I did for so many years.

If I could live that experience again, I would still invite my friend along and be there for her, but not in the same way. Instead, I would make sure I was having a good time as well. Everyone would be fine with this, including the friend I took along, who would have to manage her anxieties around strangers. And my old friends would enjoy more of my company.

I have to keep reminding myself that I'm not responsible for others. I can be there for them but not to a point where it totally absorbs me. Understanding what's at stake in a situation like that makes such a difference and helps me move forward in any difficult situation. I have been confronted with plenty of experiences like that, so by recognizing and understanding the pattern I'd fallen back into, I was able to see the bigger picture, which would help me not to eat and drink in an unhealthy way every time I felt uncomfortable. This power of being mindful, of being aware of your own behaviour and understanding the reasons for it, is not only incredibly liberating but gives you the confidence to keep on your chosen path and not regain the weight you've lost.

We live in a world where we have to always be better, do better, do more exercise, make more money, be slimmer . . . and so on. We tend to judge ourselves through the eyes of others by comparing ourselves to the people (real and virtual) around us, often imagining how they perceive us. All of this is human nature and, believe me, everyone of us has the same anxieties about the same kinds of things.

The problem is that in this constant quest for perfection we often can't just enjoy who we truly are, or savour the good things around us and the best aspects of our life. Making changes and accepting that we are good enough doesn't mean we remain the same: we can still learn new things, discover new places and find a life balance that suits us better, but it will happen organically. We can then be more mindful, and more curious about the things around us.

By now you and I will have connected via our shared experiences and through the various psychological processes I have discussed in this book. We will have explored some of your issues, and I will have explained where they came from and how they have affected you. Ultimately, I will have taught you the most effective coping strategies. Armed with this information you will learn how not to blame others anymore and become fully accountable for your physical and emotional hunger and how you satisfy it.

A greater goal than the weight loss itself is to make peace with yourself – your true self – and maintain a better image of yourself, in a kind and loving way. Just like I did, you too can reprogramme your mind, tune into your emotional and physical connections with food, and be happier and healthier than you've ever been.

Best of all, you can finally be free of all the years of negative emotions surrounding your relationship with food and continue to be healthy and happy for years to come.

I wish you every success.

Philippe x

RESOURCES

Here you will find a week's worth of the Food and Emotions Diary featured in the book, along with some blank Notes pages. Feel free to use these pages to chart your own experiences and remind yourself of the key points. Refer also to page 265 for a list of useful websites and further reading.

MONDAY	Food and Drinks
Morning	
Noon	
Afternoon	
Evening	

Emotions and Context	Hunger/Satiety/Pleasure

TUESDAY	Food and Drinks
Morning	
Noon	
Afternoon	
Evening	

Emotions and Context	Hunger/Satiety/Pleasure

WEDNESDAY	Food and Drinks
Morning	
Noon	
Afternoon	
Evening	

Emotions and Context	Hunger/Satiety/Pleasure

THURSDAY	Food and Drinks
Morning	
Noon	
Afternoon	
Evening	

Emotions and Context	Hunger/Satiety/Pleasure

FRIDAY	Food and Drinks
Morning	
Noon	
Afternoon	
Evening	

Emotions and Context	Hunger/Satiety/Pleasure

SATURDAY	Food and Drinks
Morning	
Noon	
Afternoon	
Evening	

Emotions and Context	Hunger/Satiety/Pleasure

SUNDAY	Food and Drinks
Morning	
Noon	
Afternoon	
Evening	

Emotions and Context	Hunger/Satiety/Pleasure

Notes

Useful Websites and Further Reading

Here is a list of resources that you may find useful as you embark on your new life to rediscover the real you. And do feel free to reach out to me via my website and tell me how you are getting along.

- My website: *www.philippetahon.com*

- BMI healthy weight calculator: *www.nhs.uk/Tools/Pages/Healthyweightcalculator.aspx*

- Alcohol advice: *www.drinkaware.co.uk*

- For psychotherapy tools you may be interested in reading more about the work of Eric Berne, Friedrich S. Perls and Virginia Satir, who specialize in Transactional Analysis, the Gestalt Approach and Family Therapy.

- Marriage guidance: find yourself a good therapist if you feel the need to address issues in your relationship or try any of the marriage guidance websites, including Relate at *www.relate.org.uk*

- Mindfulness: there are so many apps, downloads, books and other media available but I do recommend mindfulness expert Jon Kabat-Zinn and his book *Mindfulness for Beginners*. You can find out more at *www.mindfulnesscds.com*

- General therapy advice: *www.goodtherapy.org*

INDEX

ACKNOWLEDGMENTS

My many clients have inspired me to write this book, and I want to thank them for that. Throughout the thousands of hours that I have been working with these men, women and teenagers, I've discovered their inner richness. To put their minds at ease, not one of them is identifiable in this book. The names I give and the examples I set out are adapted from years of therapy sessions and – although their stories are all genuine – the details are created from their composite histories.

What is most humbling is that every one of the people I have helped agreed to share their deepest secrets with me and then followed my advice to achieve profound changes in their lives. Things weren't always easy and the road was sometimes bumpy, but they accepted their doubts and fears and moved forward to what many of them describe as freedom. I have encouraged them to be creative when considering their issues, and they have very often exceeded my expectations. I am so proud of them all.

Thank you to Sarah and Lenny for supporting their father throughout these years. Thanks to Stephanie Jackson at Octopus for believing in me. And thank you to Wendy Holden and Carly Cook for their warm and professional collaboration that helped me turn my passion into this book.

Merci beaucoup!

ABOUT THE AUTHOR

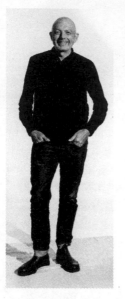

Former restaurateur and father of two Philippe Tahon switched careers and countries to become one of Europe's most sought-after therapists and weight-loss specialists. The best-kept secret of celebrities and therapists, his revolutionary approach has attracted international interest and is now available to anyone wanting to lose weight by utilizing the tools he's developed as a psychotherapist, or "shrink."

Through his contact, work and research with many health industry professionals, including dieticians, pharmacists and doctors, Philippe has discovered that, by learning to fully appreciate our hunger and the reasons why and when we eat, we can finally allow ourselves to have the body we want. He believes that unless we get to the root of the emotional and psychological triggers that devalue our self-image and urge us to overindulge, our attempts to control our eating will almost certainly fail.

As someone who gained 32 kilos (5 stone) over five years, Philippe knows exactly what it feels like to be trapped in a toxic cycle of guilt and self-loathing. Unhappy with his life/work balance, Philippe sold his restaurants, retrained as a psychotherapist and came up with his own unique weight-loss programme. This not only helped him lose all his excess weight in less than a year but, in gently reprogramming his mind to create a benevolent self-awareness, it also improved his self-esteem.

Without counting calories or going to the gym, he tuned into his physical and emotional connections with food, made peace with his body, and has remained happy and healthy since 2002. Philippe's